Everyone is affected directly by cancer in loved ones or themselves and indirectly by exorbitant cancer care costs. The **Good Fight** *reveals for everyone in intimate and inspiring detail how empowering it is to take charge of your life with cancer for both care receivers and caregivers. It is filled with practical ways to complement conventional cancer care and increase its effectiveness by shifting the focus from just killing cancer cells to strengthening your body's immune system so that it can stop the formation of cancer cells.*

—Jack C. Westman, M.D., *Professor Emeritus of Psychiatry, University of Wisconsin School of Medicine and Public Health, President, Wisconsin Cares, Inc.*

....

A wonderfully captivating, compelling, and well written story, one that clearly illustrates the limitations of conventional medicine and the remarkable therapeutic benefits of a holistic approach in treating cancer. What I enjoyed most about this book is the way in which Greg and Katherine so intimately described and applied the essence of the specialty of Integrative Holistic Medicine—the healing power of love!

—Rav Ivker, DO, ABIHM. *Co-Founder & Past-President, American Board of Integrative Holistic Medicine, Founder & Medical Director, Fully Alive Medicine, Boulder, CO, and author of the bestselling* Sinus Survival

....

The Good Fight *is a wonderful story of how love, integrative medicine and hope can lead to exceptionally positive outcomes in cancer patients. The intensely personal story leads us from the diagnosis of a rare untreatable type of cancer, to the sometimes painful process of treatment, and through to a surprisingly successful outcome. This story is worth reading by everyone who is a cancer patient or loves a person dealing with a diagnosis of cancer.*

—Paul Reilly, ND, *The Seattle Cancer and Wellness Center and co-author of* How to Prevent and Treat Cancer With Natural Medicine

....

This book is deeply moving. In a unique and powerful style, Katherine and Greg each portray their journey through painful physical and emotional ordeals few of us can imagine. With remarkable openness, they detail the uncertainties, fears and weaknesses they must confront and overcome during Greg's fight against a daunting cancer.

Many of us will some day face the abyss ourselves, or share it with loved ones, and some of those battles will not be won. But the Holmes' experience can inspire and give strength, when hope and perseverance seem so out of reach. They convincingly show how it takes so much more than just radiation and chemotherapy treatments to endure a serious malignancy. Their experience can serve as an inspiration and guide for others facing similar challenges.

—Richard M Cover, M.D.

THE GOOD FIGHT

A STORY OF CANCER, LOVE, AND TRIUMPH

To Erik —
You can do it!

Greg Holmes, Ph.D.
Katherine Roth, M.D.

PARADOX PRESS

ISBN: 978-0-615-90356-9

Paradox Press / paradoxpressbooks@gmail.com

Printed in the United States of America.

To the Memory of David Froh and Marilyn Park

CONTENTS

SUPPLEMENTALS

The descriptions of the diagnosis and treatment of cancer in this book are intended for informational purposes only and should not be used as a substitute for medical advice. The reader should not rely solely on information provided in this book for their own health problems, nor view the book as an endorsement of any treatment, clinic, or provider. Questions or concerns about your own health should be directed to your own physician or other knowledgable healthcare provider. Some of the names in the book have been changed.

PROLOGUE

ON DECEMBER 23, 1971, President Richard M. Nixon officially declared war on cancer with his signing of the National Cancer Act. In the ensuing 42 years, more than 16 million American men, women, and children have lost their lives. Approximately 1,500 people die each day in the United States from cancer.

Despite small areas of progress, cancer continues to kill us at an alarming rate. The probability is extremely high that you, or someone you love, will have cancer. On April 1, 2004, Katherine and I declared our own war when I was diagnosed with a rare and deadly cancer. I was lucky to have married a gifted physician who truly loved me and relentlessly strived to keep me alive. Katherine spent hundreds of hours researching alternative treatments not only to fight the cancer, but to protect my body from the devastating effects of chemotherapy and radiation. But the doctors we consulted dismissed Katherine's suggestions of complementary medicines, no matter how well researched. And they refused to give me hope. Any hope at all.

While I was dying from cancer I made a simple vow. I promised that if I lived, I would do everything I could to help others fight cancer. And in the spirit of hope, this book is a down payment on my vow.

−Greg Holmes

LOVE IS A CORE INGREDIENT OF HEALING but is often confused with infatuation and magical thinking of how the other will complete us. In reality it has so much more to do with making choices and taking action for the growth and fulfillment of the other. Love is a discipline.

My learning the discipline of love wasn't just in my relationship with Greg. It touched many other facets. There were moments when I confessed in the privacy of my own heart that I didn't always like sick people. Well, I didn't, but I did. My patients sought me out as their doctor when they needed help to do the things that they couldn't do for themselves, like when they gashed their hand or their baby was ready to be born. It took love to do the things for them that they could not do for themselves. How else could I place a needle to draw their blood or numb their wound? And more than physical pain, there were those times when they needed a port in the storm to prepare to do the work that only they could do—like stop drinking or change their life. I learned to listen with love.

I came to understand that the way in which one helped made all the difference. If I "fixed" you, that meant I carried the power. But if I "served" you with compassion and knowledge, I strengthened the healing power within you. Greg's illness and our relationship inspired the awakening of my servant's heart.

Yes, love is a core ingredient of healing. But so is will and spirit. The question is, do you want to live?

We cannot know when it's our time to die. But I believe that if you don't try—really try—to live, the chances of surviving are much less. We must not back down from the seriousness or complexity of what is being asked of us. We need to do everything in our power to create a body where cancer cannot thrive.

The world is ready for a more comprehensive approach to cancer. We must demand more care of the environment and more cautionary research about the use of chemicals, pesticides, and herbicides. Our goal should be to prevent cancer from beginning in the first place.

Not a single doctor we worked with during Greg's illness has ever asked me what we did to fight the cancer, but I believe many people are hungry for a more holistic treatment. We must respect the healers who are working to find ways to use natural substances, along with chemotherapy and radiation, to make treatment less toxic and more effective. I encourage anyone with cancer to seek out people who are passionate and knowledgeable about this growing area of research.

—Katherine Roth

PART ONE

"No one can confidently say that he will still be living tomorrow."

—Euripides

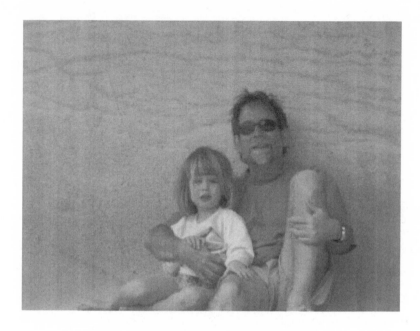

Greg and Emerson in New Zealand, 2/26/04.

1.
APRIL FOOLS

GREG

ONCE UPON A TIME I had it all: a firmly rooted marriage to my soul mate, Katherine, an exuberant three-year-old daughter, Emerson, and a lakefront home in northern Michigan. It was an idyllic life, a true-life fairy tale. Little did I know that in 2004 those halcyon days would suddenly come to an end.

April Fool's Day began to unfold just as other days had that year. The crisp, early spring morning offered no hint that it would be the day that would change my life forever. Katherine and I were awakened too early, as usual, by the small, 20-year-old GE clock radio that sat on the oak dresser. The newscast on the local public radio station was depressingly familiar; a sputtering economy, a war with no end in sight, and political bickering between two talking heads that were more alike than either was willing to admit.

The lone bright spot in the news was the weather forecast. The brutish northern Michigan winter was finally in retreat, defeated once again by the warm winds of spring. After a night of precious little sleep, Katherine and I rushed about that morning, readying Emerson and ourselves for the day ahead, one we had no reason to believe would be much different than any other.

It felt comforting to be back in the predictable rhythm of our daily schedule. The three of us had recently returned from a three-week vacation to New Zealand, and coming home was a welcome relief.

NEW ZEALAND HAD BEEN A DREAM destination of ours for many years, and we set sail for those magnificent islands accompanied by great expectations. The last film in the "Lord of the Rings" trilogy had just been released, and everything New Zealand was all the rage. However, during our trip we were faced with a small, yet persistent, frustration. I suffered for several weeks prior to the trip with a stubborn sinus infection that completely sealed off my left nostril. Katherine and I tried everything we could think of to unblock it. First, I used a simple, over-the-counter decongestant. No luck—still plugged. We thought that I might be having an allergic reaction, so we tried an antihistamine. That didn't work either. I still couldn't breathe out of that nostril!

We decided to turn for help from my internist, Dr. Kalat. He was a rarity—a kind, unhurried physician who truly seemed to care. His first love appeared to be golf, as his small examination room came complete with a putter and golf ball. On one wall was a poster of a Scottish lad with a bag full of clubs that said, "Free Golf While You Wait." Dr. Kalat methodically recorded the history of my symptoms and listened sympathetically as I recounted our failed attempts. He ordered an x-ray of the obstinate sinus, which the radiologist deemed to be "negative." Dr. Kalat concluded that the blockage was due to a simple bacterial infection and prescribed a course of antibiotic treatment. Believing that we were finally on the right path and that the worst was over, we packed our bags and took my stuffy nose to New Zealand.

The infection proved to be an extremely annoying travel companion, one that demanded our constant attention. The antibiotic didn't work and the stubborn nostril remained blocked. I became so frustrated that I tried on several occasions to blow the unwelcome intruder out of my nose. Finally, during a sunlit day high atop a breathtaking fiord on the north shore of the South Island, I closed off my right nostril with my right thumb and blew with all my might. A huge amount of green gunk poured out, and, eager to identify the perpetrator, I caught it with my bare hand. What was most striking about the foreign goo as it sat glistening atop my hand was its jelly-like consistency. It was a green slime that quivered in my outstretched palm.

As disgusted as I was by the nauseating gunk, I was also elated. Finally we were getting somewhere! I showed the glob to Katherine, who was similarly encouraged that we were making some progress. A family physician herself, she examined the unwelcome trespasser and believed it to indeed have the color and consistency of a bacterial infection. She suggested we attempt to treat it with a different antibiotic. We found a family doctor in the seaside town of Cormandel who agreed with our diagnosis and prescribed an antibiotic she was confident would fix the problem by the time we returned home. I left her modest office believing that we finally found the cure for my nose and our frustration.

As we completed the last leg of our sojourn we looked forward to returning to the familiar routine of our respective lives—Katherine, to her practice; me, to the conflicted lives of my psychotherapy patients; and Emerson, to friends and fun at her preschool program.

I BID KATHERINE AND EMERSON GOODBYE on that early April Fool's morning and climbed into our aging but loyal maroon Subaru wagon. The car, as if on autopilot, followed the well-worn path from the small peninsula we lived on to my downtown office. I looked forward to early mornings and the half hour or so of peace before tackling the problems of my first patient.

I strolled across the street to a coffee shop where the baristas knew my preferences. I grabbed my medium-sized, black coffee and scanned the metallic tables with their hard, hip chairs for the coffeehouse copy of the local newspaper. As usual, John sat in his customary corner seat carefully corralling the object of my desire. He had a familiar smug look on his round, bespectacled face. John and

I always tried to be the first to grab the front page and sports section of the morning paper.

"Looking for this?" he asked in his typical self–satisfied voice as he waved the paper in front of my face with his pudgy fist. "You can read it when I'm done." Lord John continued, placing both sections of the paper on the table under his oversized elbows. "But I guess you can have this," he declared, handing me my consolation prize, that morning's *Wall Street Journal*.

His display of faux magnanimity poured fuel on the fire of my irritation. Frustrated, I grabbed the paper from him and vowed to myself that I would beat him to the coffeehouse the next day and put an end to his ownership claims.

The *Wall Street Journal* held little of interest to me. I found the seemingly endless stock and bond tables, graphs, and stories about mergers and acquisitions to be quite boring. However, I did enjoy two features in the otherwise tedious read: the movie reviews by the critic Joe Morgenstern, and the middle, or A-Hed, column on the front page of the paper, which consisted of well-written human-interest stories. These were unusual, even bizarre accounts of people doing weird things, such as toad licking, cooking road kill, and competing in the Miss Agriculture Pageant.

However, what was in the A-Hed column that April Fool's Day was no laughing matter. It was just the opposite—a compelling story about the struggles of Andy Martin, a third year medical student at Tulane University. The article described how he was diagnosed with sinonasal undifferentiated cancer (SNUC), a disease so rare that only a hundred cases were documented in the medical literature. The cancer was described as one that killed; it was an extremely aggressive and destructive illness with virtually zero chance of survival. With so few cases, there was no desire by the pharmaceutical companies to conduct research on the disease. The article described how Mr. Martin was growing cancer cells extracted from his own nasal passage in a desperate attempt to find a chemotherapy drug that would slow the progress of the tumor and prolong his life.

The account of his struggle disturbed me, and I was immediately overcome with a feeling of shame. Here I was fighting with somebody over a stupid, 75-cent newspaper that I didn't even like, while Mr. Martin was fighting for his life. How childish could a person be? I gave my ego a good talking to, and admonished myself to check it at the coffeehouse door the next morning.

My self-recriminations did not end there. I was completely embarrassed with how irritated and self-absorbed I'd become about the problems with my nose. I'd been obsessing about the fact that the antibiotic prescribed in New Zealand hadn't worked, and how, when we returned home, an ear, nose, and throat specialist discovered a polyp in my nostril. He believed it was the culprit behind the whole thing. He biopsied the polyp and informed me that I would have to undergo outpatient surgery to remove it. I dreaded the thought of surgery as it meant intravenous sedation, and I had a big-time phobia about needles. Nevertheless, I agreed to proceed. At least we would get the darn thing out of my nose and be done with it once and for all!

All this time I had been kvetching about my pesky nose and whining about someone putting a needle in my arm, there was brave Andy Martin, left on his own, sure to be in the grave soon.

A feeling of comparative gratitude finally settled over me as I finished my coffee, grabbed my backpack/briefcase, and walked across Front Street to my office. An odd thought popped up on the desktop of my consciousness. What if my earlier frustrations that morning with John actually happened for a reason? The only thing I was sure of was that it had been a humiliating lesson; one I promised I would never forget. I was the fool that April morning!

Still, there was no way that I would thank John for my lesson that day. Humility and gratitude could only go so far, and I refused to admit that I might have actually won by losing.

The A-Hed article helped me put my problems into a much larger perspective. My marriage to Katherine was thriving, and stronger than ever; I was more and more convinced each day I was one lucky guy. We loved being parents to Emerson, the miracle child given to us when we were both forty-seven. At three, she had grown into a vibrant self of her own that was both fascinating and endearing. Katherine and I were happy with the decision we'd made a decade earlier to move to the smaller, friendlier environs of Traverse City. Katherine was on the verge of breaking away to begin practicing the kind of medicine she really believed in. Most days we realized that we were blessed. We had a wonderful life, and it seemed the polyp was my only real problem. I resolved to get the dreaded IV and surgery behind me and stop my whining.

KATHERINE

ON A FIRST DAY OF APRIL I pulled up to the convenience store on the edge of town for a hot cup of coffee. The hospital where I worked was just fifteen minutes away, and I savored the few precious moments of my coffee sipping ritual. Frost still on the windshield, I left the engine running and hurried inside.

The store was a welcome throwback to the family grocery store, and came complete with a few lonely vegetables, packaged meats, and basic hardware supplies. Rick ran the store while his elderly but spry father puttered around the periphery, keeping a watchful eye on all the comings and goings. They greeted me heartily as I dashed inside from the bitter cold. After our usual playful banter, I left the store with coffee in hand, the door swinging shut behind me.

My mind was already shifting into its work mode as I geared up for a day of doctoring and teaching. Suddenly I stopped in my tracks. What? My car was gone! I looked all around for it, but it was nowhere in sight! I searched my memory; where had I parked it? Then it dawned on me—oh my God, somebody had stolen my car!

After seemingly endless moments of gut-wrenching disbelief, Greg popped out from around the corner of the store, doubled over in laughter and looking quite pleased with himself. He had arrived at the store moments earlier and quickly moved my car to the back of the store. My feeling of initial shock quickly changed to utter annoyance, but finally gave way to irrepressible laughter. We stood for a moment in the icy parking lot, stomping our feet to stay warm and savoring our silliness. That was how I had always remembered April Fool's Day—until 2004.

SINCE THE BEGINNING of the year, I'd watched Greg struggle with sinus congestion that refused to improve. It was such a common symptom. I treated people every day with congestion due to colds, allergies, and I've even removed an occasional stone placed by curious toddlers into their nostrils. But Greg's congestion seemed different to me, and it weighed on my mind. How could something so simple be so resistant?

We tried everything: neti pots, eucalyptus steam, echinacea tea, decongestants, antihistamines, steroid sprays, and antibiotics. Even the tincture of time failed him. I encouraged him to return to his local doctor while I phoned a physician and friend Rob Ivker in Denver, Colorado, who was an expert in sinus disease and the author of *Sinus Survival*. He offered both concern and sympathy, and suggested that the congestion might be due to a yeast infection, which would have eluded antibiotics. We rallied our enthusiasm and started a medication and diet that would kill off a chronic yeast infection. Still, there was no improvement. One simple clear breath continued to elude him.

I was equally worried, if not more so, about Greg's increasing frustration and preoccupation with his congestion. The man I knew (and adored) was generous, fun loving, and optimistic to a fault. We had been together fifteen years and often debated the question of whether the glass was half empty or half full. There was no debate really.

Yet I, the methodical realist and wavering pessimist, would try my best. I'd bemoan the pollution of the Great Lakes and my sadness at its potential destruction wrought by invasive species. Then Greg would coax me down the steep, sandy bluffs of Lake Michigan for a swim. There we discovered the seemingly endless body of water with thousands of sparkling sunlit diamonds. We immersed ourselves in the hypnotic waves, body surfing until we were exhausted, or too cold to continue. I had to agree that 99 percent of the time, the glass was half full. With Greg by my side, there was always something to enjoy and some way to make things right. Now I often found him sitting on the edge of the bed, lost in a shroud of thoughts.

When I wasn't worried about Greg's congestion, I allowed myself to admit I was bored by it all. Wasn't there something more important to think and obsess about than a stuffy nose? I mean, really. The next day though, feeling a little shamed by my annoyance, the worry reappeared.

WHEN WE RETURNED HOME from our trip to New Zealand, I immediately called Dr. Noorgard, the local ear, nose, and throat specialist to get help for Greg. I attempted to remain casual as I described Greg's symptoms, but Dr. Noorgard sensed my desperation. The bottom line was, we needed more information and direction, and we needed it now. To my relief, he offered to see us the next day.

On March 30, Greg was the last patient of the day. We perched on the edge of our chairs in the empty waiting room. An ancient issue of *People* magazine lay between us, and we reached over it to hold each other's hand. Greg's was damp and cold. He had been stoic for months, but now he was openly distraught.

The nurse escorted us to the exam room where we met Dr. Noorgard and poured out our story while he listened and took notes. Then he examined Greg's nasal passage with his endoscope and quickly pronounced that he could see a fleshy polyp on the left side. He asked me if I wanted to have a "look." I hesitated, not as a fellow doctor, but as Greg's wife, but ultimately I peered through the scope. To my relief, all I saw was a smooth pink plumpness. This was no monster, no bogeyman. I reached for Greg's trembling hand and sent him my best reassuring smile. Dr. Noorgard felt confident it was most likely a benign polyp that could be surgically removed. But he threw us off when he asked to take a biopsy ... just to be sure.

Panic flashed in Greg's eyes. He had a disabling fear of needles and blood that I could never calm with reason or sympathy. Yet, he mustered up his best adult self that day and agreed to proceed. The biopsy was quick, and within minutes it was over. Shaken but relieved by our encounter, we collected our things. At last we had an explanation for Greg's misery! I went ahead to pick up Emerson while Greg scheduled a CT scan and surgery date. As I left, I kissed his still cold cheek.

THE NEXT DAY, APRIL 1, I woke early and went to my small desk. I frequently wrote in the morning stillness, pondering my dreams and meditations before the busyness of the day stripped them away. That morning I thought more about Greg and his blocked sinus. A spiritual teacher once told me that our partner was our true mirror and reflected to us our life issues. Could my difficulty with my medical practice—my blocked initiative—have anything to do with his nasal blockage? I wondered if there was any connection between the two? What work did we need to do that was so intimately linked? I realized that to help him I needed to listen more deeply.

I wrote with urgency and uneasiness about my dream from the previous night. It felt odd, like a premonition. In the dream Greg and I were at a reception, eating food that was generous but not nourishing. When we returned home, I broke out in hives that no one else could see. Greg and I began arguing, and we didn't even know what we were arguing about! He said he needed to leave, and I pleaded with him not to go, but he insisted and left. I was alone. As the dream continued, we were in a car with Greg's father driving, and his mother beside him in the front seat. I was sitting in the back with Brenin, my 19-year-old son from my first marriage, and Emerson. We were going somewhere important and the air was heavy with sadness. Brenin turned to me and observed that Greg "had such a feminine side." What unnerved me was that he said it in the past tense.

As I wrote down the dream I became scared. Was Greg's soul leaving me? For the first time, I thought of the possibility of Greg dying. A strange urge to get up from my writing desk, run to him, and tell him he didn't need to die flooded over me. Instead I stayed glued to my journal and wrote, "What he needs is for me to trust my intuition, my wisdom to assist him in his recovery. I am strong. I can listen, and when I know, I am fearless." I rose from my desk to meet the day. Like a warrior, I was ready for whatever lay ahead.

Several hours later, I was driving west across town with Emerson. She was happily munching on a cracker and we began singing a song she loved about a bumblebee. At the end of the song the child squishes the bee and sings, "Won't my mama be so proud of me?"

Suddenly my beeper went off, putting an abrupt end to the merriment. I pulled over and dialed the number on my cell. I immediately recognized Dr. Noorgard's voice. I could hear agitation in his voice, and I steadied myself with a deep breath. My heart was beating rapidly.

"Katherine, we got the biopsy report back and I wanted to get back to you as soon as possible." He paused. I waited. "It looks like Greg's polyp is actually cancer." I paused for a moment before saying anything. Had I misunderstood him? My mouth went dry and the world around me began to recede. I asked him to start over. Suspended in the vacuum of the phone call, I heard his voice repeat that the biopsy indeed showed cancer. I spoke again, this time desperately asking if this was an April Fool's joke. He paused, and gravely said, "I wish it were."

In a rush of words, he explained that he had spoken with the hospital pathologists, and they believed it was a very rare cancer. They were sending it to Mayo Clinic for a second opinion. He had already contacted the University of Michigan and arranged a consultation for Greg with their surgical ENT (ears, nose, and throat) Department. He said something about how there had been a cancellation, and they would be able to see us next week. I thanked him for his efforts, and somehow wrote down phone numbers and dates. I felt sick to my stomach. Despair settled into my body like a heavy fog.

I could barely remember my errand. Wasn't I going to drop off my time card at the hospital? As I lifted Emerson out of her car seat, I pulled her defenseless, innocent softness to me. I pressed my tear-streaked face into her body. Confused, she asked, "What's wrong Mommy?" She was the first person I would tell, but she was only three and could not understand the words I uttered: "Daddy has cancer."

A walking casualty, I stumbled across the street with Emerson in my arms. I remembered my disturbing dream and then forced it away. All of a sudden Greg's life became a fragile, precious treasure; like a mirage it flickered before me. I was not about to let the darkness of the dream take away the life I carried in my arms, nor the one in my heart. I needed to call Greg!

THERE IS SIMPLY NO RIGHT WAY to tell a loved one that their deepest fears are indeed true. I resented being told the disturbing news by Dr. Noorgard on the phone. Why hadn't he called us over to his office and told us in person? Now it was up to me to deliver the news to Greg. How could I, a quivering mess, remain strong and gentle?

I found a quiet room in the hospital's administration office and placed Emerson beside me. I closed the door and dialed the number. Greg answered the phone. For one moment, I let myself savor its warm resonance. I loved the sound of his voice despite the congestion in its vibration. I hesitated, as one does when facing a huge precipice. I knew that telling Greg would make it real and send us free-falling into a nightmare. I longed to hold back and return to our innocence. But reality pushed me forward. I asked Greg if he was sitting down, and then I jumped. I don't remember how I told him, or the words I chose, but each one felt cruel. Each word was irretrievable, shattering our world and life as we knew it. Nothing remained except the harsh, wind-swept shoreline of our tentative future.

GREG

WHEN I ANSWERED THE PHONE, Katherine sounded as if she was in a state of hysteria. The extreme sense of urgency in her voice sent a chill through my body, and I knew immediately that some horrible disaster was unfolding. My nervous system went on red alert, and my body tensed as I braced myself for the bad news that was sure to follow.

For most of my life I'd lived in fear of getting "the call"—the one that would inform me of the death of one of my parents or sisters. The fear was well founded in a painful reality after years of watching family members struggle with life threatening, debilitating illnesses. I'd spent my life in the constant shadow of my mother's various diseases: lupus, kidney failure, heart arrhythmias, and near fatal reactions to medications. She had been hospitalized on several occasions during my childhood and teen years, and I was told more than once that she "might not make it this time." My father was diabetic, had barely survived two heart attacks, and had recently undergone treatment for prostate cancer. My youngest sister, Amy, struggled with serious complications from her cardiomyopathy and the powerful medications she took for that disease.

So which one would it be? It could be any of them. But what really frightened me was the sense of urgency I heard in Katherine's voice. It was not the gently compassionate tone someone uses when they are breaking the anticipated news of the death of a loved one. It was a beside-herself voice of sheer panic, a voice of someone losing control.

"Are you sitting down?" she asked.

OH MY GOD! I thought, my mind leaping immediately to the worst possible scenario. No! Something must have happened to Emerson! No! Please God, no!

"Greg…" she continued, "I'm at the hospital! Dr. Noorgard paged me! He wanted to let me know that he got the results of your biopsy from the pathologist. He said the growth in your nose is not a polyp after all! It's a tumor! It's cancer!"

What? How could I have cancer? Katherine and I had been the poster children of good health for many years. Neither of us smoked, we both drank a half glass of red wine each evening, our diet was replete with organic fruits and vegetables, and we exercised routinely. We meditated, did our yoga stretches, and went off as seekers on spiritual retreats. We helped many others change their unhealthy habits and states of mind. We were *so good*!

Ironically, Katherine and I had just finished leading a support group at the local hospital for cancer patients, advising them how to change their lifestyles in order to avoid a recurrence of their disease. How was it possible that I was now one of them? There was no way!

Katherine's voice on the phone jolted me back to the present. "I can't believe it!" she exclaimed, mirroring my own thoughts.

"How do they know?" I asked.

"I asked Dr. Noorgard," she replied, "and he read the pathology report to me. It said the results from the biopsy are conclusive. It's cancer!"

"Did he say he was sure?" I was hoping for a second opinion from the same doctor. Perhaps there had been some horrible mistake, some mix-up in the pathology lab of my biopsy with somebody else's.

"He said it was definitely cancer," she repeated. She paused for a moment, and then continued with the words that would become my death sentence. "The pathologist said it was some type of rare cancer—sinonasal cancer."

Sinonasal cancer? It couldn't be! Sinonasal undifferentiated cancer! SNUC! The same cancer I'd read about that morning in the coffee shop! Andy Martin's disease! The article was so disturbing that it had remained firmly stuck on the Velcro of my consciousness. Words from the article flew through my mind, repeating over and over again as if they were blazing across the news ticker high above Times Square: RARE...WORST CANCER...AGGRESSIVE... NO TREATMENT...NO HOPE...NO SURVIVORS...DEATH... RARE...WORST CANCER...AGGRESSIVE...NO TREAT-MENT...NO HOPE...

Without the slightest hint of warning, our idyllic, it's-a-wonder-ful-life morphed into a nightmare and was racing to a tragic con-clusion. The truth was that I had Andy Martin's disease—sinonasal cancer! I became case #101 that day, and I was going to die.

2.

PRAYING FOR A MIRACLE

KATHERINE

THERE WAS NO DISTRACTION that night from our demons of disbelief, thoughts of death, and grief. Greg said he could not stay with us. He was frightened and worried about Emerson and me seeing his desperation. Yet how could we not notice the paleness in his face or feel the heaviness in his heart? Our lives had changed so irrevocably in such a few hours.

He drove off into the night, promising he would return. I didn't want to let him out of my sight, yet I knew he had to go. As I watched his car lights receding into the darkness, my aloneness magnified. Nothing could ease the pain, but then I looked into the eyes of my daughter, full of life and innocence. I reached out that night for strength and found my way to navigate through her bedtime rituals.

GREG

I WAS SO ANXIOUS that I couldn't sit still, and I paced about the house like a madman. Suddenly I realized what I needed to do. I grabbed my blue windbreaker and car keys, told Katherine I needed to go for a ride, and promised that I would be right back. As I left the driveway of our home, my goal that cloudless spring night was clear—I needed to find a church.

I have to admit that I hadn't been anywhere near a church for many years. My parents were Sunday Catholics, the kind who show up once a week to get their card punched. Catholicism was not my chosen religion; it was chosen for me. Going to catechism class on Saturdays felt exactly like what we were told purgatory would be like, replete with torture inflicted on those who misbehaved. My sins in the day were many, including the fact that I wanted to stay home on Saturday mornings. In those years, it was the only time that cartoons were on television.

Church and catechism didn't seem to make a whole lot of sense to me when I was young, but I quickly learned to keep questions to myself. During one of the Saturday classes, Sister Jean noticed that I did not finish coloring my picture of the Crucifixion, and instead was looking at two black squirrels chasing each other on a big oak tree. She rushed down the aisle and hovered over me, her large brown wooden crucifix dangling between us.

"And just what are you doing young man?" she asked. "Why aren't you finishing your work?"

"I don't feel like it," I replied. Why not be honest? Wasn't lying a sin?

"And just what do you think the world would be like if everyone did what they wanted to do?" she asked, triumphantly raising her arms to the heavens as if she just scored the winning touchdown in a football game. My classmates squirmed, anxious looks on their faces, eyes wide.

I looked up at her self-satisfied face, bracketed by the black and white habit. "It would be great!" I replied, thinking, it would be.

The complexion of the nun's face changed suddenly from a pasty I've-never-even-been out-in-the-sun hue to a violent, why-you-insolent-little-son-of-a-bitch red. Yet she didn't hit me that day— physically, anyway. Instead she pummeled me verbally with, "Just wait until you face Our Father! Because. Children. Like. You. Go.

To. Purgatory! If you don't listen to me and change your attitude right now you will end up in Hell!"

Religion was always difficult for me to swallow, especially the inevitable part where your religion was the one and only one that God recognized. It seemed to me that if God only wanted us to do one thing, and not have any choice in the matter, then that's the way we would have come out of the box.

Despite my skepticism towards organized religion, I had an emotional connection to many of the teachings attributed to Jesus, as well as others. I was the first to admit that I didn't have a clue what happened after people died, but I did believe that there was some being, some energetic force, or something behind the scenes. I thought death would be like going to Oz, where I would finally get the chance to pull back the curtain and find out, once and for all, who or what was behind the whole thing.

On that spring evening I was ready to accept any spiritual port that could offer me sanctuary. I was on the verge of a nervous breakdown, and I could not bear to have Katherine or Emerson witness my coming apart. It would be painful enough for them to see me waste away and die over the next few months. There was no way I could control the cancer, but I needed to find a way to "die with dignity," whatever that meant.

As I drove down a dark, two-lane road toward town, I came across a large illuminated green cross set high against the pitch-black sky. Saint Patrick's Church was a twice-a-day sight on my way to and from work, and I would often notice the oversized cross suspended above the entry. I vaguely recalled that Saint Patrick was a slave in Ireland who escaped to Great Britain and later returned to Ireland as a bishop to lead the Irish people.

The three or four cars in the large parking lot that night gave me hope that the church was unlocked, and to my great relief, it was. I was met in the vestibule by a larger than life, gold statue of Saint

Patrick, no slave to anyone now. My trembling hand opened the heavy wood door to the nave. I saw a group of people down on the far left of the church, standing around an organ, perhaps getting ready to practice for an upcoming service. I veered off to the right, went into a pew, removed my windbreaker, and immediately lost what little control remained of my emotions; I began to cry. Normally, I would have been embarrassed to cry in front of anyone, but what was happening to me was anything but normal. The dam broke, and a torrent of tears poured out, intermingled with muffled sobbing.

As I was on my knees in the pew that night, I thought of the character George Bailey, from my favorite movie, *It's A Wonderful Life*. The movie spoke directly to me as a great reminder of love, helping others, and gratitude. I'd seen it so many times I had memorized the story, and that night at St. Pat's I thought about George Bailey on the bridge, going out of his mind, contemplating suicide. George prayed, "God…God…Dear Father in Heaven, I'm not a praying man, but if you're up there and you can hear me, show me the way. I'm at the end of my rope. Show me the way, God."

I felt at the end of *my* rope, but I didn't want to jump off a bridge to save my family from shame and humiliation. I didn't want to die! My mumblings between fits and starts of sobs that night at the church went something like this: "Please don't let me die! God, help me—please! Please don't let Emerson and Katherine suffer! I can't take it…Please don't let me die! Please don't let me die! Please somebody help me! Please!"

Suddenly a hand came out of nowhere and gently touched my left shoulder. I jumped, startled out of my desperate prayer. I lifted my head out of my hands and turned around to see who it was. No, it wasn't Clarence or anyone else who identified herself as my guardian angel. The hand belonged to a woman parishioner who had been practicing with her group in the corner of the nave. In her other hand was a box of Kleenex. "Would you like one of these?"

Her compassion seemed genuine. "Can we help you?" she queried, her soft brown eyes gazing down at me.

I struggled to catch my breath, and quickly tried to explain everything in a quivering voice: that I had a bad cancer, that I was going to die, and how I couldn't bear the thought of leaving my wife and three-year-old daughter. As I was blubbering another woman came across the dimly lit church to join us.

"Don't I know you from somewhere?" she inquired. A look of recognition instantly crossed her face. "That's it!" she exclaimed, as her memory kicked in. "You shop at the food co-op and bring your daughter there to have lunch!"

Hearing the word "daughter" spoken out loud removed the few remaining screws that were holding me together. Completely unhinged, I sobbed uncontrollably. The nave began to spin, and the words of the two women standing two feet from me sounded like distant babble. "Cancer…physician…his poor daughter!" I felt as if I were dying right then, and that I was leaving my body. If this was what dying was like . . .

"Here. Drink some of my water," the younger woman offered, taking a plastic bottle of water from a green tote bag. "Would you like to see if we could get the priest? Maybe he can talk to you."

I didn't know what to do, but as I sipped the water I knew what I didn't want to do, and that was talk to any priest. The last time I talked to a priest was when I was in high school. My girlfriend's mother was beside herself when her daughter, Mary Ann, a purebred best of show, wanted to date me, a mongrel. A mongrel with shoulder-length hair, a scraggly mustache, and the audacity to park his rusted-out, piece-of-crap VW bug with a peace sign in the middle of their newly paved, circular drive.

Mary Ann was upset when her parents ordered her not to date me. Her constant arguing led to her parents suggesting they settle the matter by having me discuss the issue with their family priest.

With no option but to agree, I dressed in my Sunday clothes, thinking this would impress him. But there was no impressing the priest that day as we sat face to face in his drab office. I discovered he had little interest in finding out who I was or how I felt. Instead, he pronounced that Mary Ann's parents were right, and it would be a sin to disobey them (and now, of course, him).

"And one more thing," he snarled, "and that is about you having the long hair of a girl and the mustache of a man. You obviously have some conflict about your sexual identity." He rose abruptly from his chair. He was done and so was our meeting. "I want you to think about that. And, when you are ready to talk honestly about it, we can make another appointment. Now go in peace."

So it came to pass that I never, ever wanted to talk to another priest. I didn't make my pilgrimage to Saint Patrick's that April night to talk to a priest; I went to the church to speak directly to the source and pray for a little more time here on Earth. I went to pray for a miracle.

KATHERINE

GREG RETURNED LATE THAT NIGHT and crouched beside our bed. He took my face in his hands and, with an intensity I had not seen in months, said, "Never blame yourself! Don't ever blame yourself. You didn't do anything wrong! I love you. I will love you forever!" I made no reply, but begged him to come to bed. Somehow we fell asleep, sobbing and trembling as we held onto each other for dear life.

The following day I awoke at sunrise without an alarm. I could hear Greg's heavy breathing beside me. The memory of the previous day flooded over me. I needed to get up, but my mind had lost its ability to set a direction. How was I going to manage to see a full day of patients at the office? What were we going to do? Greg's consultation with the specialists in Ann Arbor was a week away, but it felt like months to my anxious mind.

I remembered Greg's words from the previous night: "Never blame yourself!" He knew me so well; that was exactly what was lingering behind my grief. I was a seasoned doctor. How could I have missed this? I was haunted with unanswerable questions. Why didn't we insist on a CAT scan earlier? I knew an x-ray was not adequate for the diagnosis of softer structural problems. Why hadn't we seen the ENT doctor sooner? I wondered why he'd never had a headache or a nosebleed? I'd never even heard of sinus cancer! How could that be? And then I remembered how everyone else thought it was just a nagging sinus problem—an allergy, an infection, or a common polyp. In self-defense, I reminded myself that several respected, well-trained doctors had examined Greg and had also missed the diagnosis.

All that was true, but easing my blame did nothing for my broken heart.

GREG

WHEN I WOKE THE NEXT MORNING, I turned my head toward the clock radio on the bedroom dresser and wondered how much time I had left. Six months? Maybe a year if I were "lucky"? All I knew was that the sand was running out of my hourglass.

My sleep had been fitful, interrupted by a recurring nightmare that had been haunting me over the past several months. The dream invariably began with a jet making an emergency landing in an odd place, like the parking lot of a mall or a cornfield. Terrified, I would start running to the crash site while trying to call 911; yet I was never able get anyone on the phone. My anxiety over the situation would become so unbearable that I would wake up, startled and drenched in sweat.

I've always been fascinated with dreams; they were the reason I became a psychologist in the first place. Originally I'd wanted to become a lawyer, and I began a prelaw curriculum at Michigan State University. During an introductory psychology class I was introduced to the hidden world of the unconscious by a brilliant, eccentric professor. One of our assigned readings was Freud's seminal work, *The Interpretation of Dreams*. I was astonished to discover that there was a whole other world that existed, one that was just a free association or two away from our awareness!

I was hooked. Someone else would have to be the next Perry Mason. I returned home during spring break and announced I was now going to be a psychologist instead of a lawyer. My mother's face looked like she'd bitten into a lemon. "A psychologist," she said. "Well, just don't start psychoanalyzing me!" She wasn't kidding. Nor did she realize that it was way too late.

Years later, after working with many patients, I'd became increasingly convinced that dreams were extremely significant and potentially invaluable. Dreams reveal the unconscious, and when analyzed in therapy, can often be the key to unlock emotional conflicts. Recurrent dreams were the demanding children of that other world, pushing the dreamer over and over and over again to pay attention to their message, a message that was often difficult to decipher.

The mechanical malfunction in my dream that night sent the jet heading for a crash landing. However, this time I wasn't on the ground, watching the jet crash, trying to contact the police. I was on the jet, and I was screaming.

I jumped out of bed. The sheets were soaked. I was terrified. I finally understood the meaning of the nightmares. The dreams had been trying to warn me that I was going to crash, and now it was too late. I was losing altitude, fast.

Terrified, yes, but I wasn't about to give up—not yet anyway. Maybe I'd watched too many movies where the pilot was somehow able to pull the plane out of a nosedive at the very end or stop the train before the tracks ran out. I couldn't stand still and watch myself crash!

I dressed, put on my game face for Katherine and Emerson, and resolved that I would go to work and concentrate on my patients. I decided not to tell anyone about my cancer. The last twenty-four hours felt like a hallucination. I wanted to wait and see what happened at our visit to the University of Michigan before facing anyone with their questions and concerns.

KATHERINE

I SAID GOOD MORNING TO THE STAFF when I arrived at my office, yet I was numb to their cheerfulness. Over years of doctoring, I had learned to empty my mind of personal concerns while attending my patients. I would literally forget the details of my own life as I listened and became immersed in their lives, fears, and the nuances of their stories. Today this was impossible. I saw my first patient and knew I was in trouble; I was completely preoccupied. There was no way I could distance myself from our family's painful reality. I could barely remember what to ask or how to proceed through the simplest visit.

Finally, there was a midmorning break. A patient had rescheduled and the exam room was empty. I went immediately to the phone and called the radiology department. Greg's CAT scan had been done on March 31 and the report should be dictated by now. I spoke to the receptionist, and navigated the questions that would allow me access to the report. Then I hesitated. Did I really want to know the results?

Suddenly, I understood my dad's desire to deny the dysfunction and illness of our family and retreat into the sanctuary of his recliner with *The New Yorker* magazine. I saw how tempting it was to cling to some earlier, easier version of today. But even though I might want to, I could never do it. My love and desire to help Greg propelled me forward.

I picked up the faxed report. My eyes raced over the page. I read the words "large soft tissue mass"…"Areas of bony expansion, bone erosion and bony destruction"…"5 cm mass involves the nasal cavity…involves the left maxillary and sphenoid sinuses in their entirety"…"The cranial fossa…eroded or destroyed with upward convex character." My heart was frozen as I held my breath. "Oh my God!" It was much worse than I had imagined. Our nightmare became even darker.

My associate, Sharon, came into the room, and in a torrent of words I explained to her what was happening. I handed her the report. Her intelligent, professional face revealed it all. She looked as though she were reading a death sentence. I saw disbelief as her mouth parted with a small gasp. She confirmed what I could barely perceive through my panic. Greg was desperately ill; he was close to death. I put the paper down with a trembling hand. How could I return to the exam room and face my next patient?

I opened the exam room door and discovered a good friend, someone who had known our family for years. She took one look at me and asked, "What's the matter?"

Without warning, I broke down and sobbed, trying to utter the words to describe Greg and his illness. I don't know if any of it made sense. I knew I was breaking all kinds of professional rules. I shouldn't be disclosing my personal problems to a patient. Where was my capacity to compartmentalize? I didn't know and I didn't care.

Slowly I regained my composure and managed to get a hold of myself, redirect the visit, and care for her needs. She gave me a generous hug as we said goodbye and I softened for a moment. The day wore on and on. Walking through the shadow of death, I somehow found a way to move one foot in front of the other.

That evening, standing at the kitchen sink, I heard Greg's car drive into the garage and I stopped what I was doing as the door opened and closed. What would I give for one ordinary day where I could look casually over my shoulder and welcome him home? I vowed if there ever were such a day, I would run to him, as I was running now, and embrace his dearness. In that moment, I understood Einstein's insight that it was the wise person who saw the miracle in the ordinary.

Now it was my turn to take Greg's face in my hands. I asked him questions that I had never allowed myself to ask anyone in my life. "Why is this happening? Why do we have to go through this? Why you? Why us? Why now?"

We looked at each other with unwavering eyes. I didn't expect an answer; that wasn't what I needed. I needed to find my voice, and I needed to ask the questions. What was happening to him was happening to me. Our compass needle had shifted, and for whatever reason, as horrible as it was, we were being sent down this uncharted path—one we had never imagined would be ours.

I asked the unknowable, but doing so allowed something to shift. It was time to stop falling apart and to start responding. My familiar childhood feelings of victimization, hopelessness, and powerlessness began to recede.

Later that night, as we fell into merciful sleep, another dimension reached out to me and rode beside me. I felt the intelligence of the universe, witnessing and present. I had felt its presence before in my life when I faced major challenges and changes. It was as though my desire was magnified through a force other than my own; it wanted me to find my way as earnestly as I did. It was like being in a shadow theatre, with me on one side of the curtain and the life force shimmering and shining through on the other, collaborating, facilitating, reciprocating. I believed the power given from this other dimension was in direct proportion to the effort we put forth here, on this side. I knew my effort would be there. Greg's life depended on it.

GREG

THE SHOCKING NEWS OF MY CANCER set Katherine and me off on a panic-driven scramble to find a lifeboat on our sinking ship. Articles on the Internet about SNUC confirmed the bleak reality described in the *Wall Street Journal*. The disease was indeed a rare, very aggressive and fast growing cancer with no reports of survivors over five years. Stories of "treatments" for sinus cancer were horrifying. Surgery, even if possible, was extremely disfiguring as the surgeons entered the sinus area by cutting down through the top of the head or up through the jaw to remove the tumor. The best outcome from this gruesome procedure was to slow down its progression, but in the end it would only delay the inevitable. We held on to improbable hope that the doctors at the University of Michigan would know of a new treatment and could get me into a clinical trial.

I was no stranger to the hospitals at the University of Michigan; I'd spent two years of my doctoral training in Ann Arbor. One year I was on a long-term diagnostic unit for very disturbed children and adolescents, many of whom had committed serious crimes. Jimmy, a tall, skinny, constantly smiling, 10-year-old boy was my first patient there, and my tour guide into the psychotic world of pyromania. He never talked about his past; he preferred to act as if he came out of nowhere. However, he did like to play games and draw pictures.

One day he proudly presented a picture he'd made for me. It was a traced outline of his right hand, with violent red flames shooting out of all five fingertips. Even though he never acknowledged his past, the thick chart in the nursing station said it all. Jimmy had been strung up repeatedly from the pipes on the basement ceiling as a young boy and whipped with a belt. Psychosis was the only sanctuary in his abusive home.

During my second internship, the patients were older, and the violence they had witnessed was overseas. The veterans in the VA hospital described the unspeakable events they had both witnessed and committed in Viet Nam. Like Jimmy, they lived their present lives through the filter of a tortured past. At times it felt like I was trying to pick up a bunch of Humpty Dumptys, and neither I nor the king's men could put them back together.

Now, more than twenty years later, I was heading down the road once again to the U-M hospitals, this time as a patient—a Humpty Dumpty in my own right. True, I hadn't had the crackhead boy-friend of a teenage mom whip me, or the Viet Cong shoot at me... My killer wasn't hiding in the basement of a dilapidated house in a Detroit slum or slinking through leech-infested rice paddies of Asia...My enemy was inside me. My enemy was me.

My feelings of panic were all consuming. The confirmation that I was sick and dying of cancer crashed through whatever walls of hope and optimism I tried to construct. I choked back tears each time I looked at Katherine and Emerson. What had they done to deserve something like this? I remembered the uncertainty I had lived through as a small boy struggling to cope with my mother, who seemed to be always on the verge of dying.

If it were just me who was going to die—well then okay, I guess, if I have to. By the age of fifty, I more or less had come to accept that everyone has to die someday. But that "someday" had seemed so far, far away—a good thirty years away—in my eighties, maybe.

I was painfully aware that no one ever dies alone; that an irreplaceable part of those who survive also dies. I knew from working with grieving patients that you never "get over" your loss; the best you can do is to learn to live with it. I began to imagine Katherine and Emerson's lives without me. Katherine would be a grief stricken widow and a single mom trying to raise a little girl who, in all probability, wouldn't be able to remember her own father. I knew Katherine would remember how much I loved her, but what about little Emerson, just three years old? Was it even remotely possible that she would remember me? I couldn't remember a single thing from my early years—I could barely even remember where I was the day that JFK was shot, and that's when I was ten! I sobbed quietly into my pillow and made a vow that I would tell both of them, each and every day, how much I loved them; that I would continue to love them forever.

3.
GOING FOR BROKE

KATHERINE

GREG WAS DYING. The awareness of this interrupted me count-less times throughout the day, and I would quickly bury it with the retort, "Don't think that!" I truly believed in the power of thought and refused to accept that he might die. I couldn't imagine living without him.

Everything came to a standstill in our lives. Everything. What else really mattered? Work, food, sex, movies, even my spring garden—they all paled in the harsh light of Greg's condition. We were lost in our own thoughts as we prepared for the next step, whatever that might be.

Emerson was the only one who didn't change. Her chubby hand in mine calmed my racing heart. We listened to her favorite Rafee CD with songs of a mother duck quacking after her ducklings that had flown away. She danced to the lyrics with Pink Bear, a stuffed animal and constant companion. She loved wrestling with Greg on the queen-sized bed, rustling the comforter and sheets into a total mess. They would roll around and cry out as though they were on some dangerous precipice and then fall off the bed onto the floor, laughing.

Emerson was our best medicine. Her songs and the games played out our own fears of separation and danger, yet it was the laughter and the surrendering to the present moment that saved us.

Still, I couldn't shake off the numbness and surrealism. The disconnection to my feelings was frightening. I needed a safe haven where I could feel what I was trying so desperately not to feel and to talk to someone who wasn't directly involved in our lives. I decided to go into town to see my friend David, a gifted body worker and healer.

As I lay on my back in his exam room, looking into the emptiness of the darkened ceiling, I began to put words to the events of the last few days. Tears streamed down my cheeks. In the silence, I prayed, "Let my heart stay open. Let me feel."

David massaged my shoulders and sobbing chest, and spoke to me of "manifested prayer." He explained that often when we pray we end up focusing on all that is wrong in our life. Instead of guiding our consciousness in the direction we desire, we become entrenched in the problem. He suggested I simply envision fully what I wanted to see happen—in every single detail.

My thoughts turned to what was foremost in my heart. I saw Greg, vibrant and strong, looking back at me with his twinkling blue eyes. He was with me, relaxed, happy, and healthy, and we were celebrating the opening of my new practice. There was no hesitation or doubt. My heart broke wide open and I felt peace rush in and fill the space beside the pain. I returned home that afternoon and began to prepare for our trip to the University of Michigan.

THE CONSULTATION IN ANN ARBOR was just a week away, but I knew we needed to begin his treatment now—but how? I wondered how long the cancer had been there. Cancer is made up of thousands of cells, but it begins as one malignant cell that divides, and then each cell continues to double. Each doubling usually takes a month. It can take 30 doublings of the cells before it grows to one centimeter. Thirty doublings would take 30 months! How long was 30 months? Two to three years! Greg's tumor was five centimeters.

How long had it been there? One year? Two years? Five? My mind reeled as I realized how long the cancer had been living with us, stealth-like, for years.

I was totally thrown off guard by Greg's diagnosis and, at first, had no idea what we were going to do. I was frightened, derailed by the rarity of the cancer and its dismal track record for survival. Greg was too young. We needed each other to raise Emerson. All of this was so overwhelming.

Yet within 24 hours I sat bolt upright in my bed and urged myself, "Wait a minute! You have to move through the fear and despair! You don't have the luxury to second-guess yourself! You need to do something. Deal with it!"

Wasn't I a doctor, after all? I was much more equipped than 99 percent of patients and their families. Was I going to just sit around and wait for the specialist to decree what we already knew? Even the *Wall Street Journal* was aware of the crappy prognosis! Was it really true that there was nothing else but traditional cancer therapy? After years of studying holistic approaches that included nutritional supplements, and honoring the role of food and herbs as life-saving medicine, I knew the answer. There was a lot to be done!

The first book I turned to was, *How to Prevent and Treat Cancer with Natural Medicine*. The lead author was Dr. Michael Murray, whom I had personally met when I invited him to Traverse City as part of our Integrative Medicine Speaker Series. We had emailed and spoken with one another on several occasions. The other contributing authors, Dr. Birdsall, Pizzorno, and Reilly, worked in cancer centers that combined traditional chemotherapy with a naturopathic approach. Their real work in the trenches offered not just theories of how things worked, but precise doses and frequencies of supplements. I trusted these doctors and the information they had painstakingly researched and shared.

I had referred to the book frequently when developing and facilitating a cancer group at the hospital. There it was, on my desk forever overflowing with articles and magazines. I pushed everything else aside and dove in. Information that just days before was remotely interesting was now critically important. I needed to save Greg's life. Nothing could distract or deter me. My hungry eyes returned to the book again and again, studying it whenever I had a free moment or a sleepless night.

I knew that nutrition played a key role in both the development and treatment of cancer. I devoured every sentence on how nutrition and supplements would not only lessen the damaging side effects of radiation and chemotherapy, but could actually increase their effectiveness. I vowed to create a program that would work synergistically to improve Greg's survival.

THE GOAL OF CHEMOTHERAPY is to destroy rapidly growing cancer cells, but the problem is that it cannot differentiate cancer cells from healthy cells. Both are destroyed simultaneously. Particularly vulnerable are cells lining the intestinal tract, the mouth, hair, and the developing red and white blood cells. Side effects from chemo typically include nausea, vomiting, mouth sores, and an overwhelming lack of appetite. It soon becomes a struggle for the patient to eat—anything.

I bit my lip as I read about the loss of appetite and the wasting away process of the body known as cachexia. It could even occur in people who were eating enough, but were unable to absorb the nutrients in the food. The tumor released chemicals known as cytokines that increased the body's metabolism, accelerating tissue breakdown and exacerbating the cachexia. Their disease-ravaged bodies became like a bucket with holes in it. My mouth dropped open when I learned that 40 percent of cancer deaths were not from the cancer itself but from the effects of malnutrition!

KEEPING THE DIGESTIVE TRACT FUNCTIONING

With chemotherapy and radiation causing breakdown of the lining of the GI tract, it is extremely important to actively work to help it repair and stay healthy. Further insults occur if you are on antibiotics, NSAIDs (like aspirin, C elebrex or mobic) and a diet of refined carbohydrates with low fiber.

Things that I gave to Greg (or added to his shake) included:

- Probiotics including lactobacillus and bifidobacterium (25-100 billion organisms)

- Saccharomyces boulardii, a probiotic especially useful if you have antibiotic-related diarrhea or possible yeast overgrowth

- Glutamine is an amino acid that is critical to the repair of the lining and feeds the cells of the entire GI tract. Work up to 3 grams three times per day.

- Zinc 30-60 mg per day, critical for the immune system and wound healing

- Coconut oil or milk is loaded with MCT (medium chain triglycerides), a source of fuel for your cells. It also discourages yeast and viruses. It can handle high temperatures so use it on hot cereal or in stir frying vegetables.

- Gentle Fiber such as ground flax seed or arabinogalactans (500-5000 mcg). Arabinogalactan stimulates NK (natural killer cells) and blocks the metastasis of tumor cells to the liver.

- Keep sugar to a minimum. Strongly consider a gluten-free diet.

Using antioxidants during chemotherapy is controversial. Some of my research sources were the following:

- Today's Dietician, 2010 (http://www.todaysdietitian.com/newarchives/040510p26.shtml)

- Integrated Cancer Therapies, 2006 (http://www.aminomics.com/pdf/Antioxidants%20%26%20chemo.pdf)

- National Cancer Institute, 2008 (http://www.ncbi.nlm.nih.gov/pubmed/18505970)

- National Cancer Institute, 2009 (http://www.ncbi.nlm.nih.gov/pubmed/19141775)

- Integrated Cancer Therapies, 2005 (http://ict.sagepub.com/content/4/4/271.refs)

I didn't need anymore convincing of the importance of what I could provide Greg. I just needed to *begin*, but where? Greg didn't even take a daily multivitamin, and from my reading and research, there was a growing list of nutrients that he needed.

I started him on high quality multivitamins with minerals, along with extra high doses of antioxidants; vitamins C, D, and E; probiotics; and fish oil with omega-3 EPA/DHA.

I was acutely aware that the use of antioxidants during chemotherapy and radiation was extremely controversial. Most oncologists flatly prohibited patients from taking them. Their concerns were that the antioxidant might protect the tumor and undermine the treatment. However, when I reviewed the research, just the opposite appeared to be true.

Cancer cells, when exposed to the appropriate levels of antioxidants, increase their rate of self-destruction (apoptosis) and are less able to switch on the genes that tell them to grow. In addition, the antioxidants protect healthy cells from damage, thereby reducing the side effects of radiation and chemotherapy. The levels of antioxidants that might theoretically interfere with chemotherapy were astronomical, and could never be reached with oral supplementation, such as vitamin E dosages of 35,000 I.U! At the levels I was prescribing to Greg, the "protection" to his cancer cells was akin to a bulletproof vest in a nuclear explosion—meaningless, except to his normal cells. I came to the conclusion that taking antioxidants at appropriate levels during chemotherapy allowed people to tolerate treatment better. And most importantly, to survive longer.

I also knew that protein was very important for cancer patients—so important that they need 50 percent more than their usual requirement to repair the immune system and build up blood supply and muscles. I began to envision Greg, just weeks from now, developing difficulty eating as the treatment progressed and the tumor advanced. I had witnessed the decimated appetites of my patients going through chemotherapy. I wanted us to be prepared for this and not flounder for weeks as so many of them did.

MUCH HAS ALSO BEEN WRITTEN about the importance of whey protein and its role in cancer therapy. Whey comes from milk, but is separated from the casein, the portion of milk that is responsible for most people's allergy. That's why it's called "pure" whey protein—there's nothing left but the protein. When compared to proteins from rice and soy, whey has the highest biological value. It's more easily absorbed, retained, and used by the body. This super protein also contains the highest amount of glutamine, an amino acid that significantly helps with the repair of the lining in the intestines, the nose, and mouth.

BASIC WHEY SHAKES

- Whey protein powder (20-30grams) plain or flavored
- 8-12 ounces of filtered water or almond, coconut water or nonfat milk
- Few ice cubes
- Place ingredients in kitchen blender and serve fresh. Reduce liquid if appetite diminishes or quantity seems overwhelming. Adjust protein powder if too thick.

Optional ingredients to increase variety/flavor/caloric content

- ½-1 cup frozen or fresh fruit
- ½ avocado
- 2-3 Tbsp nut butter
- Ground flaxseed for fiber and texture
- 1-2 Tbsp Omega 3 oil from flaxseed, may use oil from deep water fish if pure and mild taste
- Kefir or yogurt (rich in probiotics i.e. beneficial bacteria)
- Probiotic from opened capsule
- Grated ginger for tang and to ease nausea
- Cinnamon for warmth
-

Information on whey protein and its importance during cancer therapy can be found here:

- Mayo Clinic (http://www.mayoclinic.com/health/whey-protein/ NS_patient-wheyprotein/DSECTION=evidence)
- Research & Development Department, Immunotec Research Ltd. (http://www.ncbi.nlm.nih.gov/pubmed/11205219)

What really caught my attention had to do with the ability of whey to assist in the production of glutathione, an antioxidant that's present in every cell in the body. Think of glutathione as an important member of your body's clean-up crew—it works as a master detoxifier that helps rid the body of unwanted or poisonous substances. Interestingly, many cancer cells contain more glutathione than normal cells, perhaps explaining why cancer cells can become resistant to chemotherapy. The extra glutathione actually protects them!

Whey protein paradoxically reduces glutathione in cancer cells while at the same time increasing the glutathione in healthy cells. Wow! So if tumor cells were depleted of glutathione, they would become more susceptible to cancer treatment. Meanwhile the normal cells and tissues had some protection from the poisoning effect of chemotherapy! This was simply not seen with other proteins!

The information empowered me. Without question, I knew that I needed to make whey protein shakes a foundation of Greg's program. They might be a welcome alternative to the Ensure shakes that Greg had already tried and refused to drink.

Every morning I headed to the blender and varied my concoction with fresh blueberries, black raspberries, or the basic favorite, banana. I wanted them to taste good, and I kept trying to improve their palatability. Yet I could never predict Greg's reaction. It seemed the vanilla shakes with added bananas won out over the raspberry with its pink tartness. As time wore on, I stopped licking the blender or watching his face for approval. I wasn't trying to be the next Julia Childs, I just wanted to be Greg's life-saving nutritionist.

I DECIDED THE WEEKEND BEFORE our university consultation to call Dr. Robert Leichtman, a conventionally trained internal medicine physician who had slowly morphed his practice into what he really was—a medical intuitive. I explained Greg's situation carefully, then asked him for his insights. He hesitated and mumbled, and I heard some rustling. It was like turning on a radio and taking a moment to get the station tuned. He talked at length about Greg's work and his attitude toward people who didn't want to change. "He's had quite a snoot full over the years. He has come to expect more of his clients, and they show him things he just can't fix. It frustrates him. All the years of unfinished events come back and curl on themselves. They actually curdle. It's like a miscarriage, with the creative substance not being expelled. He tries too hard."

Dr. Liechtman finished his consultation with his bottom-line, "No, he doesn't have to die, but you should do absolutely everything. This is the time for a wholesale review. His cancer is five centimeters, you know. You should go for broke on this one."

From that day on his words of advice became my mantra: *Go for broke.*

Like the spider in *Charlotte's Web*, I developed a vision to save the life of my beloved friend. The outcome was uncertain, but I had to try.

I REMAINED SKEPTICAL ABOUT CONVENTIONAL MED- ICINE. What did it really know about healing? Thirty years ago, in the 1980s, there was little proof that the body had the ability to heal itself or to reverse chronic disease. One of the first pioneers in "lifestyle" medicine was Dr. Dean Ornish, who developed a program for reversing heart disease. He demonstrated that if a person ate a low-fat diet, exercised, and reduced stress, they could actually reverse cardiovascular disease. It was a revolutionary challenge to traditional medicine.

The medical community received the news with a shake of their heads, and many concluded that Ornish must be some kind of a quack. Even if it were true, who cared what the research showed if patients wouldn't do it? His multi-pronged program was like a drug—the more a person "took," the better they did. Someone might exercise regularly, but actually meditate? And what difference did it make if people began to love and make peace with themselves and others?

Dr Ornish has continued lifestyle medicine and research and turned his attention to prostate cancer. He has been able to show that diet, exercise, and meditation influenced gene expression. Specifically, by following his program, some disease preventing genes were turned on and disease causing genes were turned off.[1]

Greg and I had used this holistic approach when we created a program for heart patients at Sparrow Hospital in Lansing, Michigan, in 1992. Out of thousands of people with heart disease, we connected with just a dozen willing souls every few months. Greg, in his affable way, could put even the most uptight, Type A person at ease. He told them offbeat stories and discussed sports trivia until the patients would forget that they were in a hospital and working on big-time stuff like survival, not to mention change. I often ran late to our class, and by the time I entered the room, the assembled group would be all smiles. Greg was already there, and had told them he was just the warm-up act! He would proceed to introduce me as the Big Kahuna, or some other crazy title, while referring to himself as just a "Sherpa" or the faithful dog, Snowy, from the Tin Tin comic book adventures.

Soon our post-op heart patients were moving the heavy tables around and setting up yoga mats like we were at some Sunday picnic. I'm not sure it was what the cardiac rehab staff had in mind for "gentle exercise." At the end of each class the nutritionist would encourage them to sample tofu chili and garbanzo bean dips.

And then we talked and created a sense of community. Slowly we began to breach the questions about their hearts. What did their

---

1 Gene expression original research published in preceedings by *The National Academy of Sciences*.

hearts really want? We read poetry and talked about the wounds in their hearts. Were they broken-hearted? Was there a way they could be whole-hearted? The class turned out to be transformational for many of them, and it definitely was for us. We asked ourselves the same questions we asked them. Greg and I were on our own journey to deepening our authenticity.

GREG AND I DISCOVERED that working with people in our cancer groups was much more challenging than working with cardiac patients. The stakes were often much higher, the outcomes less certain. Once diagnosed, many people feel they have been given a death sentence, and often they are right. The grueling treatment can create as much fear, if not more, than the disease itself. Open-heart surgery is no walk in the park, but cancer therapies are toxic, close cousins to poison.

I didn't understand just how great fear was for most cancer patients. One woman with breast cancer struggled with her fear when she even thought of yoga. I discussed how it might help with her lymph edema, assisting the movement of lymph through her lymph nodes. But she worried yoga might "spread" the cancer—what if that happened when she stretched her arm up? She was frozen with fear, literally afraid to move her body.

In cancer patients the fear could spread, multiplying like the cancer cells themselves, into all spheres of their lives, including their diet. There was a pervasive concern among patients, often promoted by their oncologists, about taking anything that might "lessen the effects," or interfere in any way, with the chemo. People were reluctant to take even a multiple vitamin, and cautiously eyed the bright green broccoli that contained antioxidants. Were antioxidants actually safe? The patients in our cancer group were afraid to move, to eat, and to cry.

This was how Greg and I unwittingly prepared ourselves for his diagnosis. We had shepherded scores of patients through their disease, and now it was our turn. We came face to face with the fear, the desperation, and the heartbreak. I thought back to Dr. Leichtman's parting words. Everything was on the table...nothing was out of the question. We needed to go for broke.

4.

LAST REQUEST

KATHERINE

THE TRIP TO ANN ARBOR FINALLY CAME. We packed the car and drove downstate to a good friend's house in Okemos. They generously offered to take care of Emerson for the day while we drove another ninety minutes to Ann Arbor. Emerson seemed content in their pullout bed as we headed out in the quiet darkness of early morning.

I was eager to meet the people at the ear, nose, and throat clinic. I had spoken several times on the phone to the clinic coordinator, Patty. She was always clear and optimistic with her directions on when to come, where to find the office, and the list of people Greg would see. My mind, on high alert, zoned in on her and the reassurance she offered.

After much searching, we found an empty parking space in the mammoth parking deck where hundreds of cars were already parked. It wasn't even eight o'clock in the morning! I hesitated as I stepped out of the car with a small tote bag over my shoulder. Would I ever be able to find my way back to the car? I made mental notes in the dim light of the garage, memorizing the numbered pillars and colors of the elevator doors.

The lines on the floor and the maps were just as Patty described, and we followed the yellow one. I had been part of hospital design meetings over the years, and we often discussed how to help patients navigate unfamiliar territory. Now it was Greg and me, holding hands, trying to find our way as we bumbled through the long impersonal corridors. We began to feel intimidated by the very structure as we walked deeper and deeper into it. Finally we found the sign for the Otolaryngology Center.

I half expected to see Patty at the door awaiting our arrival. We entered a large room filled with people sitting in rows and rows of chairs. I missed the smallness of our town and the familiarity of our local hospital. We checked in with a young woman behind the counter, and learned it was her first day on the job. She seemed eager to do everything correctly, but was unprepared to meet our gaze, to make that human connection. Instead, she kept her head down as she matter-of-factly handed us a clipboard with forms to complete.

We settled into the first row of the steel-framed, maroon-covered chairs. Greg stared blankly at the clipboard and confessed, "I can't write now. Can you do this?" I removed the unwelcome task from his lap and coached him to take some deep slow breaths and to un-cross his legs. He did just as I asked, a worrisome sign.

I began filling in the details of his family history, personal history, and a symptom checklist. In the past I had often been reassured when I encountered these lists: there were so many symptoms and diseases that we didn't have. And as I contemplated the laundry list a flash of hopefulness came over me. Maybe, just maybe, he wasn't so sick after all? Then the truth returned with a vengeance. We had crossed over the line. We had become one of those people with a real illness. Insomnia, check. Congestion, check. Cancer, check. I looked down at Greg's legs and noticed that they were crossed.

GREG

WE FINALLY MET PATTY, a perky medical social worker who welcomed us with a big handshake and an oversized smile, out of proportion to her relatively short stature. "Welcome to the otolaryngology clinic," she announced, just like a greeter at Walmart. She explained that she would be our "guide" that day, helping us navigate the various consultations and exams in the clinic. She let us know straightaway that she "understood" what we were going through must be "very difficult indeed," but she was equally quick to add her reassurance that we were "definitely at the right place now." There was a cheerleader quality to Patty's enthusiasm, and it was something I needed with the time running out on my clock.

Patty went over our itinerary for the day. First I would be interviewed and examined by various members of the clinic team. Second, the team would combine the results of their exams with a review of records sent by my regular physician. Finally, our visit to the clinic would conclude with a team meeting during which the chief resident and a neurosurgeon would announce their conclusions and offer their treatment recommendations to us.

KATHERINE

GREG'S NAME WAS CALLED and our consultation began. As a physician, I encourage my patients to bring a loved one to important medical meetings. Lots of things are said very quickly in medicalese and important instructions are given to the patient. It can be invaluable to have another set of eyes and ears. Now I was that person accompanying my loved one, but I was as shocked and worried as Greg. Where was my "other" person?

Greg was carefully positioned in an elaborate chair with a headrest and foot pedals. He was questioned and examined repeatedly, his body going up and down, and up and down again as a stream of doctors came to examine him. Greg gave the same answers to the same questions multiple times. "Yes, you can stick your scope up my nose. No, I have never smoked. No, I had never been a wood-worker who worked with exotic woods." He was so vulnerable and frightened that he would put up with just about anything for help.

Fellows, residents, and medical students all lined up with their respective exam lights and scopes in an effort to catch a glimpse of the extremely rare tumor that they would probably never see again in their lifetime. Up to now they were lucky if they'd even read about it. They did their best to hide their excitement. They spoke in hushed voices and mumbled verdicts, remaining professional and considerate. As they examined Greg I could feel the abyss widening between them and us. They had their health and security; we had our disease and despair.

GREG

AT LAST, THE EXAMINATIONS CAME TO AN END and it was time for the team meeting with the doctors. Patty ushered us into a small, windowless conference room somewhere deep in the bowels of the clinic and gestured for us to take our places around the ta-ble. Her seemingly permanent smile changed into an anxious look when she saw the micro-cassette recorder we'd brought with us and placed on the table. We hoped that it would assist us in our recall of this important meeting. "It would be better if you didn't have that out there when the doctors come in" she said.

"Why?" I asked. I was confused. I explained the purpose of the recorder, and shared my assumption that it was pro-forma for pa-tients to bring such a device so they could remember everything.

Patty's perkiness disappeared, replaced by a furtive look that suggested there were more dangers than my sinus tumor lurking about. "The neurosurgeon is very uncomfortable with people recording these conferences," she explained. "He walked out of a meeting this morning when he saw that a patient had a tape recorder on the table. It's probably best that you don't have it here as it will really upset him."

Katherine and I understood the neurosurgeon's allergic reaction to tape recorders. Like many doctors, he was afraid that patients would sue him, and his words would come back to bite him in court. He was covering his ass. As a top neurosurgeon at a major hospital center, he didn't need us the way we needed him. We dutifully packed the tape recorder away along with any objections we had.

Patty's ebullient mood returned instantly. "The doctors will review all your tests and results, and will be here in just a few minutes," she said as she left the room.

Those next "few minutes" seemed like a few days. As I sat in the chair I hoped and prayed that the conference would be different than I feared. The fact was it did turn out to be different than I expected—it was much worse.

The meeting was called to order by a tall, blond-haired doctor who was just a few weeks away from completing his chief residency at the clinic and on his way to a faculty position in Florida. He began the meeting with an announcement that the nervous neurosurgeon would not be attending my conference after all. The surgeon had reviewed the CT and PET scans of my head and summarily dismissed my tumor as "inoperable" because there were not enough "margins," or space, between the tumor and the other critical things in my head.

The chief resident went on to present a summary of the findings from our day in the clinic. The multitude of tests and exams only served to confirm the grim conclusion already reached at our local hospital; I did indeed have SNUC and there was no known treatment for it.

He shook his head as he fumbled back through my chart. He said he had no idea what caused my odd cancer—the few case studies that had been reported in the medical literature mentioned a possible link between SNUC and working with exotic woods.

"But don't worry," he continued, quickly regaining his footing with a more familiar self-confidence. "We're going to attack this tumor, hit it with a combination of radiation and chemo and shrink it down, and then we'll go in and we'll get it! And we don't go in like this," he said, taking his hand and shoving it up against his upraised jaw like a cocked gun. "We go in like this!" He finished his enthusiastic demonstration by raising his gun-hand above his head and pointing his index finger down toward the scalp area above the left eye. He seemed quite satisfied with his plan of attack. "Patty will make the arrangements for you to see the oncologist and radiation oncologist and get it all started." Patty, back in cheerleader mode, vigorously nodded her agreement as the doctor left the room.

KATHERINE

I KNEW A SURGEON NEEDED TO HAVE "MARGINS." Greg's cancer was too closely positioned to everything that mattered—his eyes and ears, his brain. The tumor was so large there was simply not enough normal tissue to give the surgeon the "space" he needed to operate and be confident the tumor was completely removed.

Greg was in tears, and I was close behind. We were like a mis-filed letter that had slipped through the wrong slot. What did all this mean? What were our options? It was Friday, and the day was growing late.

The chief resident said he needed another biopsy of the tumor for a second opinion from the hospital pathologist. We didn't expect this, and I could sense Greg's reluctance. At the same time he was desperate to do whatever was necessary, and he gave his consent. He pressed his back against the exam chair and crossed his legs. The biopsy was one more injury to the man I loved. I held his hand and fetched him a Styrofoam cup of water.

I felt powerless standing there, watching. Suddenly I realized that Greg needed to take some MCP (modified citrus pectin) immediately to prevent any possible metastasis during the biopsy. A biopsy can inadvertently release cancer cells into the blood stream. MCP is a dietary fiber derived from the peel and pulp of citrus fruits, and it binds to cancer cells and interferes with their attachment to each other. It can prevent cells from clumping together and spreading to other parts of the body.

Greg needed MCP and he needed it now! I explained to Greg that I was going to get something from the car. I left the room and ran down the clinic hallway while begging my stressed-out mind to retrace our steps to the car in the ten-story parking deck. To my amazement, I was able to find the car and the MCP powder that I had brought with us. I raced back to Greg, who was sitting alone in the procedure room, holding a white bandage across his face to control the bleeding from his nose. I steadied my shaking hands as I mixed the MCP powder into his cup. It was like Alice in Wonderland. *Drink Me! Work some miracle in this crazy world!*

GREAT LINKS FOR MODIFIED CITRUS PECTIN (MCP)

- http://www.faim.org/newfrontiers/modified-citrus-pectin.html

- http://www.dreliaz.org/modified-citrus-pectin-makes-chemo-safer-and-stronger/

- http://www.lef.org/magazine/mag2009/mar2009_Modified-Citrus-Pectin-Fighting-Cancer-Metastasis-Heavy-Metal-Toxicities_01.htm

Important discoveries continue to be made about this substance and support using it long term rather than just at the time of surgery. It has been found to block galectin-3, a sticky cell surface molecule that allows cancer cells to aggregate and metastasize. Other important findings include its ability to make chemotherapy more effective. Because of its multiple mechanism of action, it is an important adjuvant therapy even in the most treatment resistant cancers.

Recent research:

- http://www.newswise.com/articles/new-research-modified-citrus-pectin-a-potent-anti-cancer-therapy

- http://www.cancer.gov/cancertopics/pdq/cam/prostatesupplements/healthprofessional/page4

MODIFIED CITRUS PECTIN DRINK

- 6 grams MCP powder
- Dissolved in 2-4 ounces of water or Juice twice daily

To ensure absorption MCP should be taken on empty stomach

Especially important to take prior to procedures, biopsy or surgery

Best to take 3-7 days prior to and following procedure. Harmless and with little to no side effect and may be taken indefinitely.

Consider taking first and last thing of the day. Like all fiber, it should not be taken with medication. Take 4 hours after last dose of drug so your body will benefit from both MCP and medication. Be creative with timing.

GREG

KATHERINE HURRIED OFF, leaving me to ponder the chief resident's approach. *Don't worry*—was he serious? I hadn't thought that it was possible to sink any lower in my mood that day, but I was wrong. There I was, under attack by a vicious killer tumor, and he tells me not to worry? How did he think that was even possible? His militaristic, Top-Gun demonstration scared the hell out of me! He admitted earlier in the conference that no one knew the first thing about how to treat my cancer. Now he was ready to attack something he didn't even understand! I knew for certain then what I'd only suspected before: there was a lot more to worry about than my cancer.

SO IT ALL BOILED DOWN TO THIS: chemotherapy and radiation were the only "options" offered that day, and each one came with the certain guarantee of pain, a promise of toxicity, and the probability of hastening my death.

Patty left the conference room momentarily to check on something. Katherine leaned toward me, grabbed hold of my hands, and asked me what I wanted to do. I didn't hesitate for a second; it was crystal clear what I wanted to do: I told Katherine that I wanted to fight.

"Fight?" she asked. "How?"

"Fight!" I answered. "Fire with fire!"

Katherine gently squeezed my sweating palm. We scanned each other's face, and, as allies, began to plan our war strategy. We knew that my cancer was aggressive and already attacking me. We needed to respond with an equally aggressive counterattack, and we agreed to throw everything and anything at the tumor.

I told Katherine I thought we should accept whatever chemo and radiation options the Cancer Center could offer, and begin treatment as soon as possible. I knew Katherine was already hard at work researching and selecting nutritional treatments for our arsenal.

Our strategy session was interrupted by a soft knock on the door. It was Patty, holding my already bulging patient file. "Have you come to any decisions?" she asked in a lilting voice, much like a car salesman asking a customer about their choice of color and upgrade options for their new car. But there was no choice of color for our mood that day; it was coal black.

We told Patty that I wanted to go ahead with the chemotherapy and radiation, and I wanted to start the treatment now—like right now. This request seemed to rattle Patty, and her confidence was momentarily shaken when we veered from the typical protocol. She fumbled as she tried to regain her footing. Well…she just didn't know…that might not be possible…she would have to see…people were very busy . . .

We tried to ease her angst by suggesting that she call and "just see" if it was possible to start that day. We explained it was difficult to go back and forth to the Center as we lived four and a half hours away and needed to make daycare arrangements for our three-year-old daughter.

Patty left the room, and after several minutes returned with "some good news." She was able, after all, to get me an appointment that afternoon with the oncologist, Dr. Francisco, a specialist in head and neck cancers who would supervise my chemotherapy. I asked Patty if chemo and radiation ever cured anyone with my type of cancer. She quickly assured me that it did, and gave an example of a young man who was diagnosed with a sinus cancer "years ago" and was able to return to his work as a rehabilitation therapist. "Every once in awhile, when he has a recurrence, he just comes in and we take care of it—just like that," she said, snapping her fingers. I asked Patty if the man's cancer was the same type as mine. "Well, come to think of it…I'm not sure what type it was. But don't worry; we help a lot of people here. Our doctors are some of the best in the world."

I didn't find Patty's optimism reassuring or her confidence contagious. But I grabbed her words and guzzled down the small sip of hope they contained, much like a man gulping a thimbleful of water after crawling through a scorching desert.

KATHERINE AND I WERE LIKE A SMALL WAVE on vast sea of cancer patients. Of course, I knew that cancer was ubiquitous, that it affected the lives of millions of people each year. Prior to that day the most cancer patients I had seen at any one time were ten when we ran our cancer support group. The other 11,999,090 people with cancer that year were hidden from my view. The disease, once distant and in the background, now jumped to the foreground and swallowed me to the point where I could see or think of nothing else.

I wondered how differently I would have been treated if I wasn't married to a physician. Would I have been able to get an appointment at the clinic so quickly, or would I have had to wait for months while my cancer ate me alive? What about seeing an oncologist the very same day that we decided to go ahead with treatment?

I felt an odd mixture of gratitude and guilt when I thought about the millions of people who did not have ready access to health care: the poor people without an advocate to help navigate the system, and the uninsured. I wondered how many people died waiting for treatment.

KATHERINE

GREG'S DECISION TO PROCEED WITH CHEMOTHERAPY that day shocked me. I thought we would go home, talk about it, and carefully weigh the pros and cons. No. Greg was determined in a way I had never seen before. He was ready to walk across a bed of red-hot coals. I could see it in his eyes. He was not about to stop and weigh the odds.

This was not the man I thought I knew, the one who hated needles and tests, the man who was anything but impulsive, the man who openly complained about being confined by his seatbelt. However, I did know that he was masterful in transitions and in his sense of timing. He certainly was that day! His eyes flashed with a mixture of grit and grace. He implored, "Katherine, I want to live. I will do whatever it takes to make that possible. Help me." When he said he wanted to "fight fire with fire," I knew exactly what he meant. I nodded my head, and in my heart I promised to do whatever I could for him. I would carry him through the desert on my back.

When Patty returned with the resident, I looked once again at Greg. He held a bloodstained bandage to his face while balancing a stack of medical records on his lap. Patty gave a simple directive for our journey. Follow the orange lines. I pushed Greg's wheelchair through the labyrinth of interconnecting hallways, down a set of elevators, and through an underground and strangely empty corridor. All I knew with certainty was to keep my eyes on the orange lines. There was no past, and there was no future. We traveled up a ramp, through several sets of double doors, and into a new waiting room. Finally, the nurse called Greg's name. He was the last patient at the late hour of the day.

GREG

KATHERINE PUSHED ME THROUGH the large metal frame doors of the Cancer Center where we were greeted by a sickening sweet smell that reminded me of my grandmother's house. No cleaning agent in the world can disguise the odor of impending death. My chest tightened as soon as the automatic doors clicked shut behind me. The cancer had trapped me, and there was no escape. It felt like I was being taken to my cell on death row.

I realized then that I was afraid that I would never come out of the hospital alive, that I would die there, as my dear friend Marilyn had four months ago. Marilyn had been one of my very best friends. Over the years I'd become convinced that she was the personification of Pollyanna Whittier, the small town heroine of the book *Pollyanna*: like Pollyanna she was always sunny-side up, invariably believing that everything would work out for the best, grateful for what she had. It wasn't that she was naïve, she just didn't poke around looking for the worst in people. She had a profound, sincere innocence that I found both captivating and inspiring.

Illness had been a difficult partner to Marilyn for much of her life, and I believed that was one reason why she liked to stay up late at night and ponder the meaning of it all. She devoured books by self-professed psychics. Television programs that described near death experiences and past lives enchanted her. Our discussions would often continue deep into the night as we pondered The Big Questions. One such night, after partying a bit too much, we sat together in her hot tub, searching the starry sky above for clues to "it all." She suggested we promise each other that whoever died first would agree to find a way to let the survivor know what "the other side" was really like. I guffawed in response—was she kidding me? She didn't flinch as she repeated her proposal.

Not long after our promise, Marilyn fell seriously ill. She was ultimately diagnosed with polycythemia vera, a blood disorder. Her bone marrow produced too many red blood cells, and the disease began to take its toll, eroding her body over the next several years like the constant, pounding waves that eat away the lakeshore. She and her husband spent many grueling months searching for answers that never came. Her doctors ended up removing her enlarged spleen, and administered anticancer drugs in a last ditch effort to regulate and stabilize her blood.

But there was no answer, no cure. Her health deteriorated, and she was finally admitted to the University of Michigan hospital. And now here I was, a scant four months later, at the portal of the same hospital! I slumped down in my wheelchair as I remembered how Katherine and I had sped down the road on a panic-stricken trip to Ann Arbor to see if we could help Marilyn during her last days. I'd been scared; I knew that she was very sick, at the edge of death. I'd watched her health deteriorate over the years, feeling impotent. I so badly wanted to believe that Katherine would come up with some new idea that would save her once we got to the hospital. I was aware this was wishful thinking, but I just couldn't accept the fact that one of my very best friends was dying.

Now it was my turn. I wondered when—not if—I would be admitted, and which room I'd be in when my grief-stricken family surrounded my bed as I took my last breath. Would I die in the same room that Marilyn did? In the same bed? Would she turn out to be my tour guide to the "other side," beckoning me toward her in a tunnel of blinding white light? I didn't look back over my shoulder as we entered the Cancer Center—I couldn't. Somehow, I knew if I did, I would jump out of my wheelchair, run like the dickens, and never come back.

WE ENTERED THE CENTER ON LEVEL B2, checked in at the registration desk, and were given directions to the clinic where my oncologist's office was located. There were 150 oncologists spread out over several different clinics that were organized by tumor types. Every floor of the enormous center was jam-packed with patients, some still able to walk without assistance, many with various forms of disfigurement, each one wasting away.

Dr. Francisco's office was located in a small, nondescript cubicle at the center of the complex. Like most doctors' offices, there was an overall feeling of sterility to the space. There was no art on the bland walls, no windows for fresh air that might bring life inside. Dr. Francisco's medical student and resident, who were rotating through the clinic, met us in the waiting room.

KATHERINE

AS I LOOKED WEARILY around the antiseptic room I realized that our psychic reserves were exhausted. The oncology resident walked in, and from the tone of his voice and the pace of his questions, I knew the young doctor was tired too. I had been there. Throughout my medical training, there were never set work hours. You stayed until the last patient was seen, their orders dictated, the lights turned off. We were the unwanted additions to an already busy Friday afternoon clinic. As we told our story one more time, I realized the separation between Greg and me was gone. I too had this terrible cancer.

GREG

ALTHOUGH THE RESIDENT ASKED THE SAME QUESTIONS I had already answered three times that day, I was determined to be patient with the seemingly endless process. I understood that I was at a teaching hospital, and that the students were trying to learn the fine art of diagnosing and treating cancer.

My mind began to drift as the nervous resident wrote down my well-rehearsed responses. For many years Katherine and I had tried to teach uninterested family practice residents the fine art of interviewing patients. Our efforts proved to be largely a waste of time, as we discovered that only a third of these future practitioners showed a caring bedside manner. The rest were unreachable. It seemed they hid from their vulnerabilities and feelings behind thick, fortress-like walls of arrogance. They acted as if they didn't need anything from anybody, especially someone trying to teach them "touchy-feely stuff."

My patients were often incredulous that I could "sit all day and listen" to them. True, it is difficult to sit still, hardly moving a muscle while focusing intently on what is said, while guessing what is unsaid. If you cared for your patients, you joined them on a bipolar roller coaster ride of their emotions. Your mood would rise up with their victories or drop when they suffered tragedy. Many doctors avoid getting emotionally involved with their patients. It's simply too difficult.

I cautioned my patients not to expect an abundance of compassion or sympathy from medical specialists when they went for their consultation. I encouraged them to see the specialists for what they really were—highly trained technicians whose job it was to try to help them solve a puzzle.

So I didn't expect a lot of hand-holding from Dr. Francisco that day, or some sort of Kumbaya experience. Yet, he proved a pleasant enough young fellow who introduced himself by his first name. He was tall and slender, fussy in dress and manner. He told us that he'd reviewed my records and discussed my case with the resident. His conclusion was the same as all the doctors before him; I had an extremely rare and deadly cancer.

KATHERINE

DR. FRANCISCO DELIVERED HIS UNSURPRISING VERDICT and explained there wasn't much known about Greg's cancer. We sat in stillness; the hush in the room was deafening. There was so little left to ask. We were now in the "algorithm for unusual undifferentiated cell tumors." The doctor broke the silence by describing the different combinations of "chemo cocktails" that were available. In his opinion, Greg's tumor was best treated as a small cell lung cancer. He recommended adjuvant chemotherapy with Etoposide and cisplatin in an attempt to shrink the tumor and sensitize it to radiation.

I realized then the day had turned to night. I thought of the world somewhere outside these bleached walls where the sun was setting golden red. I longed for us to be part of that world. I closed my eyes.

Meanwhile, Dr. Francisco explained that Greg would be discussed at next week's case conference, a meeting of mixed disciplines—oncology, surgery, and radiology. They would put together their best approach. A strange mixture of relief and unease filled me. Greg was a "case"—an uncertainty. Dr. Francisco expediently wrote the prescription for the chemo, as well as an order for another

PET scan. We expressed our desire to begin the chemo immediately, and he said he would have his staff call upstairs to make the arrangements.

There was unspoken tension in the air. Greg asked about his chances for survival. Would he live? Dr. Francisco hesitated. His guarded professionalism rose like a flag, waving in the windowless room. "We don't really know the percentages of the five-year survivals. There are just too few numbers." His hollow words hung in the air.

GREG

DR. FRANCISCO SHOOK MY HAND and wished me good luck. I managed a feeble smile and muttered thanks as Katherine pushed my wheelchair out of his office. I needed more than luck. I needed a miracle.

We left his office and headed across Level BI towards the chemotherapy infusion clinic. As we passed other clinics I saw hundreds of patients accompanied by their loved ones. I imagined their trials and the pain they experienced during their treatment. A young boy screamed at the top of his lungs, "No! No! No!" as his mother dragged him toward a treatment room. Why did cancer have to attack him? We were in the middle of a war with an enemy that was killing hundreds of thousands of innocents each year!

I felt just like that little boy and wanted to scream too as we passed through the doors of the infusion clinic. I was as scared of the upcoming IV as I was of the toxicity of the drugs. Needles of any kind were my lifelong nemesis. I have always dreaded the very thought of getting a shot or having my blood drawn. I am well aware that my fear of needles is unfounded—a true phobia. Sometimes I would get so nerved up, my eyes would begin to tear as I sat in the phlebotomist's chair, waiting for the invariably young woman (does she really know what she's doing?) prepare a silver tray with color-coded tubes and the damnable syringe.

I trace my fear of needles to the doctors who I felt had lied to me about my childhood shots. Sometimes they would call it a "little prick." Other times it was sold as "just a little mosquito bite." No matter how they spun it, every time it turned out to be a big fat lie. How can you trust people who lie? I've come to believe over the years that losing trust in someone is an awful lot like losing your virginity—once it's gone, it's gone.

It was incredibly embarrassing for me to admit to my fear of needles to the phlebotomists who drew my blood. I was supposed to be the psychologist who was on top of such things. However, my honest confessions were always met with great sympathy, followed by well-meaning but unsuccessful efforts to convince me that my fears were normal. I appreciated their efforts, but I never felt normal. Instead I felt like I was a 51-year-old baby. There was no way I could ever watch the blood being sucked out of my arm.

As we entered the infusion clinic at the Cancer Center I saw 30 or so gray, Naugahyde recliners that held a true melting pot of America: people rich and poor, black and white, Latino and Asian, young and old, all forced by cancer to sit side by side while a chemo nurse administered the steady drip of chemo "cocktails."

My nurse ushered us through the human mosaic into a separate adjoining room with a hospital bed and various monitoring equipment. The nurse explained that my first infusion would be observed closely to see how I "handled" the treatment. She squirted a cold, gooey gel on several areas of my chest, stuck small white discs onto the goop, and snapped wires from the heart monitor onto the discs. The monitor emitted a steady beat, but I didn't need to look at the dancing green lines on the small screen. I could feel my heart racing.

Two clear plastic bags hung on opposite sides of a thin, stainless steel rack beside my hospital bed. My nurse explained which chemo drug was which, but I hardly heard a word she said. My attention was riveted instead on the IV syringe, coiled like a rattlesnake on the silver tray beside the bed. She asked me how I was doing, and I replied honestly that I was scared. She tried her best to comfort me as she inserted the needle, and the IV eventually found a frightened vein. The infusion pump began its slow rhythmic pulse. The fight was on.

As the chemo began its death march through my veins, Katherine grasped my hand and we looked deep into each other's eyes. Now my body was under attack by two deadly foes—the terminal cancer and the poisonous chemicals. How could I ever survive this two-pronged assault?

KATHERINE

WE MOVED AS IF IN A DREAM. A name tag was placed on Greg's wrist. It was difficult for me to watch as they hung the first bag of cisplatin and connected it to his IV site. I thought of his precious life and healthy cells meeting their first, punishing wave of chemotherapy. As hard as it was to be a patient, it was also miserable to stand by and watch. As the IV drip, drip, dripped each drop into his veins, I prayed to find some way through the treatment.

Greg looked at me from the white-sheeted bed. He asked if I could close the drapes of the windowed treatment room. Then he reached for me with all the passion and intensity of a person who knows that life is short and so worthy of living—and enjoying. I hesitated at the audacity of his longing for me in this crazy place. Then it dawned on me that this might be the sanest thing we could do...and the most courageous.

GREG

IT WAS AN OUTLANDISH IDEA to be sure, yet I remembered that even prisoners on death row are granted a last request before they are executed. I didn't want a steak dinner that day, I wanted to be as close as I could to Katherine. It was not enough to be on the same page with her; somehow I knew we needed to fuse our energies into one incredible force.

We asked the nurse if we could have some "privacy" and not be interrupted. Katherine reminded the nurse that she was a physician, and promised to watch me carefully and call if anything went wrong during the infusion. My nurse agreed and left the room, closing the door behind her. Katherine climbed up on the bed, navigating her way through the high-tech jungle of plastic IV tubes and monitor wires. Our bodies formed a spiritual double helix as we sent our love, hopes and dreams into each other.

MY MIND LEFT THE HOSPITAL and returned to that magical night on Maui when we'd raced together aboard a small sailboat named *Cinderella* into a blazing sunset. Just as the sun fell into the sea, the majestic full moon began its steady climb over Haleakalā Mountain. The humpback whales that had been swimming beneath us began to play, taking their turns leaping out of the dark sea. Our youthful captain, Rosie, tossed a microphone overboard, and the giant whales, as if on cue, began to serenade us with their songs. Everything about the sail seemed perfectly choreographed: the brilliantly backlit sky; the giant, graceful dancers; the soulful singing of the Cetacean choir. We were spellbound.

Katherine and I returned to our seaside condo later that night only to discover that the show was far from over. As we lay in bed, marveling over what we had just experienced, Katherine turned toward me and whispered, "Greg, I have a feeling I could get pregnant tonight." I wanted so much to believe her, yet I knew it would be a miracle. We were in our mid-forties and had come to the conclusion that Katherine's biological clock had run out. Yet there was a mysterious energy in the air, an energy that would ultimately trump scientific probability. Katherine's clock turned out to be just like a Timex watch—still ticking. Our daughter, Emerson, came into our lives that night.

We joined our bodies in the Hawaiian Islands, and in the process, created a new life. Now it was my clock that was running out. Could we create new life within me?

A COCOON OF WORDLESS INTIMACY wrapped around us as the last drops of chemo pumped into my left arm. Katherine snuggled under my other arm, infusing me with the power of her love. The nurse came in the room, pulled the rattlesnake from my vein, and gently massaged my bruised arm.

"How are you doing?" she asked.

I looked at Katherine out of the corner of my eye. "Better," I replied. They started to help me back into my clothes. Tears of happiness welled up in my eyes as I realized I wasn't going to be admitted to the hospital that night after all. I was going to walk out the doors. At least for now, I was going home.

KATHERINE

WE DROVE TO OKEMOS IN SILENCE that April evening. We knew we could never return to the life we had known twelve hours earlier. The only way forward was to reconnect with the existence we cherished. We were going to be with our daughter and our friends, and that was all we knew. As we entered their house, we found them sipping lukewarm tea in their dimly lit family room. Emerson was sleeping peacefully in the pullout bed, and beside her was an Easter basket full of colorful turquoise, yellow, and orange eggs, waiting to be hidden and found.

I wondered if something hidden was waiting to be found within us, too. I believed, and still believe, that the body is an instrument for the soul, and that we were souls with bodies rather than bodies with souls. Greg's body was ill—frighteningly ill—and we were frantically trying to heal it. But how? Did we really know what was wrong? I mean, really? I couldn't stop myself from wondering if his soul chose this path we were on. Could his soul be trying to help him take the steps that he was here on Earth to take? Could this illness be here to help me somehow? Greg and I were once told by a psychic that we were "twin flames," and the idea resonated with us. He believed that our life purpose was intimately intertwined. Was this horrible illness here in order for us to evolve?

5.

GHOSTS IN THE NURSERY

GREG

I LET OUT A HUGE SIGH OF RELIEF as we left Ann Arbor. It made me realize that I had not taken a deep breath the whole time we were at the hospital. I replayed the events of the day and thought about what I'd said earlier, that Katherine and I needed to fight fire with fire.

Fight fire with fire? Hmm, on second thought, the words I'd voiced with such great conviction seemed foreign to me. Where had they come from? I felt like some kind of puppet dummy, and that someone else had put the words in my mouth.

I leaned back in the car seat and tried to understand where "fight fire with fire" came from. Was it a missive, some kind of internal command? As a psychotherapist I was well aware of the "fight or flight" response. When people are stressed, their sympathetic nervous systems automatically go on alert, preparing them to either engage in aggressive, combative behavior or to run like hell. But I couldn't exactly run from the killer cancer that was gobbling up my healthy cells and tissue like some neurobiological-terrorist version of Pac-Man. There was simply no escape.

The likelihood that we would defeat the cancer was nil; it was an impossible mission, one that could never succeed without some kind of miracle. I felt like I was being chased by a monstrous villain to the edge of a towering cliff, and my only choices were to jump and fall thousands of feet or be killed on the spot. I didn't have to think about it for a millisecond; there was absolutely no way I was going over without a fight. Over my dead body—literally! We were either going to kill the son of a bitch, or it would kill me.

Our decision to fight the tumor came from two of the most unlikely fighters on the planet. Katherine and I were cut from the same cloth; we were a pair of pacifists who abhorred fighting in any form. We were anti-everything violent: guns, war—you name it. Katherine was an outspoken member of the local chapter of Physicians for Social Responsibility, and, in that role, gave talks to parents, encouraging them not to buy war toys for their children.

We had both gone through more than enough conflict in our childhoods, and the last thing we wanted to deal with was more of it. Unlike many of my friends' fathers, mine never encouraged me to stick up for myself. In fact, you could say he taught me how not to fight by carefully corralling his own angry impulses behind an impenetrable wall of passivity. He managed to avoid conflict in our family by abdicating control of the household to my mother, while he escaped to the sanctuary of work in his clothing store.

Occasionally my mother sent me into the exile of my father's store. I would help out by straightening piles of slacks and sweaters and vacuuming the floor. One dreary day, we rode enveloped in a familiar silence past the diminutive shops that lined Plainfield Avenue, heading toward the rapidly deteriorating downtown district of Grand Rapids. Suddenly my father turned to me and delivered what would prove to be his life philosophy: "There's only one thing you have to remember," he said, with an uncharacteristic firm conviction, "and that is, the customer is always right."

Puzzled, I asked him to explain. Even as a young child I knew you couldn't be right all the time—wasn't that what Mrs. Goldsmith, my third grade teacher, told Jimmy just the other day in front of the whole class? So then how could customers always be right? If they knew so much, then why did they keep asking his opinion about things? And why did I have to remember they were always right?

My father dismissed my questions with a backhanded wave. "Doesn't matter," he grumbled, eyes fixed straight ahead. "All you have to remember is that the customer is always right." Later, as I peered through my tower of Hager slacks and Van Heusen shirts, I would cringe when a customer was rude to him or made demeaning comments about the merchandise. I had come to believe that my dad was a coward. He would never stick up for me or anyone else.

The only fighting ever allowed in our home came through the small black and white RCA television. My father had little use for the shows my sisters and I liked, such as *My Favorite Martian* or *Lost in Space*. "Television is a waste of time," he declared as he withdrew to his basement workshop.

But Friday nights were a different story: "It's fight night!" my father would proclaim with uncharacteristic enthusiasm as he commandeered the television to watch the Gillette *Fight of the Week*. He would sit trancelike in his old rocking chair, a generous glass of Dewar's Scotch in one hand, his pipe in the other. He would implore me to join him. "Greg look at this," and I would grudgingly accept his invitation. It was one of the few times during my childhood when the two of us were alone together.

My father's fascination with the Friday night fights was strange. When I looked over at him I saw the flickering black and white images of the boxers reflected on the thick lenses of his black-rimmed glasses. I wondered how anyone could enjoy watching two men beat the crap out of each other, especially someone who wouldn't even stick up for himself! The excited, almost manic, rapid-fire delivery of the fight announcer, Dan Dunphy, stood in stark contrast to the economical judgments made by my father as we watched the fights.

"Good fight" or "Bad fight," he would declare in a low murmur after each match finished.

My body recoiled, nauseous, as the fighters pummeled each other. I simply had no stomach for it. Mercifully, ABC cancelled the show in 1962 after Benny "the Kid" Paret died from injuries sustained during a bout. My father and I retreated safely back to our separate corners of the world: him to his clothing store, hunting, golf and drinking, me to my friends and the siren song of adolescence.

The turmoil of the 60s and early 70s only served to widen and cement the distance between us. It was a great relief to all when I bid farewell to my parents' world and departed for the Oz-like emerald pastures of Michigan State. Fate, however, demanded an encore. The Selective Service lottery of 1971 brought us back together. My birth date was one of the first ones selected and I was ordered to report for a pre-induction physical. My father accompanied me on the melancholic drive to the induction center, a ride that I felt would be our last together. I was convinced that I was on my way to certain death in Asia.

After a half hour or so driving along the billboard-littered freeway towards Detroit, he tepidly broke the deafening silence. "Maybe it won't be as bad as you think," he ventured, as if speaking to himself. "The Army was one of the best things that ever happened to me."

I held what I knew to be true in silence. As a stateside clerk he never fought a battle. He was the lucky one who enlisted to escape his terrible childhood. At the end of that day, it was my flat feet , not my dad, that saved me from the killing fields of Southeast Asia.

I successfully avoided conflict with my family during the next several years. My attendance at family gatherings was dictated by holidays and a sense of duty. By unspoken agreement, visits were kept superficial. Yet no matter how deeply I tried to bury my past in the back yard of my subconscious, my psychotherapy patients would dig it back up and faithfully drop it at my feet during their sessions.

Such was the case in 1997, when a psychiatric resident I was treating mentioned the 1996 documentary, "When We Were Kings." I couldn't understand how a film about boxing could appeal to anyone, much less an educated, caring person. I was shocked when he told me that it had won the Oscar for Best Documentary. What disturbed me the most was that he urged me to see it. "You have to see it," he said. "You will like it."

I quickly dismissed his comments as a wishful projection. A sudden chill came over me, and I wondered for a moment if I was coming down with something. I made a mental note to check the thermostat after the session was over.

Finally, I caved in and rented the video. Watching the film was strangely compelling. There was Mohammed Ali, poet laureate of the boxing world, fighting for his life and the World Championship against George Foreman, a bruising, inarticulate boxer hell-bent on destruction. Foreman's laconic meanness stood in stark contrast to the engaging, verbally acrobatic Ali. There was a vivid portrayal of their fight preparations: Foreman, isolated with his attack dog in his training camp, savagely attacking the punching bag; Ali, embracing the Africans of Zaire while jogging through their villages, lovingly chased by adoring crowds chanting "Ali, Boma ye!"

The journalists in Zaire were afraid that the fight was a dangerous mismatch and that the smaller Ali could be injured or worse by the hard-punching Foreman. Their concerns appeared prophetic in the early rounds as Ali was backed up against the ropes and took a vicious beating from Foreman. Ali had provoked Foreman with pre-fight verbal jousting, and Foreman responded in the ring with unrelenting wild rage. It seemed to the sportswriters covering the event that Ali would not only lose the fight, but also his life.

In the seventh round, the large, boisterous crowd of Africans began to scream in unison the same words that they had shouted at Ali when he'd run through their villages. "Ali, Boma ye! Ali Boma ye!" which meant, "Ali, Kill him!" Their raucous pleas appeared to breathe new life into Ali, and he answered their collective call with a lightening quick series of punches that knocked Foreman down and out in the eighth round.

I was shocked by how excited I became while watching the film. My heart was racing wildly when Ali came from behind and won the fight. My psychotherapy client was right after all. The documentary continued to grip me in a weird, hypnotic stranglehold the entire day. It was then I remembered the Friday fights with my father, and I made a quick note to mention to him that he should watch the video.

Meanwhile my father and I were engaged in a slow but steady dance of rapprochement, fueled in large part by my willingness to participate in things he enjoyed, such as golf, drinking single malt Scotch, and watching college football. I discovered that any relationship with him needed to be triangulated through those activities. During one of my monthly calls to my parents I mentioned to my father that I had seen the documentary.

"That was when Ali beat the crap out of Foreman!" my father responded, with the rare passion he seemed to reserve only for boxing.

"He really did!" I said, then tried to impress him by telling him the back-story of the fight that was described in the film.

"Yup," he said, chuckling. "Now that was a good fight."

As if there ever was such a thing, I thought. We said our perfunctory goodbyes and hung up the phone. What I didn't realize then was that thirty years later I would know exactly what he meant.

KATHERINE

MY FATHER WAS A FRUSTRATED, ANGRY MAN. When he drove us to school, he yelled at other drivers with words we weren't supposed to use. He made promises to us he did not keep, and—worse yet—forgot he'd ever made them. In first grade, I had a moment of emotional clarity and I said directly to him, "I hate you." His disbelief quickly turned to rage, and he chased me through the house. I, being the fastest runner in my class, dodged around furniture and scrambled across an empty double bed. He would not be deterred or see the absurdity of a grown man chasing his daughter to settle the score. I ran to the kitchen and hid behind my mother's skirt, as she stood at the sink. She turned in laughter, thinking we were playing. My dad, breathless, grabbed me and spanked my backside repeatedly with a hot hand. That day I learned I could and would speak my truth, but it would not be easy.

My mother became ill three years later, shattering what remained of my childhood. One summer evening, when I was eight, my father came to pick us up at the outdoor roller rink. We piled into the backseat of our blue and white Chevy. He turned to us and explained that our mother had been taken to the hospital. He said simply that she was sick and had tried to hurt herself. He mentioned something about her wrists. The air was heavy and I scooted backwards against the big seat. As I looked out the window, I trembled but I did not cry. I was filled with sadness as large as the night sky. It was my first glimpse into the world of psychiatry and the hide-and-go seek of my mother's mind.

I know something about not fighting. I know, for example, that lying down in the midst of despair is not a good strategy for me. I tried that once in the summer of my tenth year. My parent's marriage was unraveling and we were the captive bystanders. My brother retreated to his room, and my sister, a young teen, disappeared somewhere with her friends. I stood between my towering parents and pleaded with them as they argued. Couldn't they stop and listen to one another? The juice glass breaking against the wall was their answer. My mother resented that her husband wanted her to drop out of law school, didn't approve of her work with the migrant workers, and had no desire to discuss the human soul. He wanted the children cared for, dinners cooked, and the linen closet orderly. It was an untenable arrangement and a gnawing pain settled inside me.

That summer I would lie down on the sofa hoping to stop the growing ache in my stomach. When my mother sat beside me, the cushion sagged a little, and the pain grew stronger. The summer day passed and I was moved to the only air-conditioned place in our one-story ranch house—my parent's bedroom. It was a haven of escape from the humid heat. The quiet, the coolness, and the hum of the air conditioner comforted me as I listened to the coming and goings of my family. Days passed. I couldn't eat, and it became difficult to even drink.

We didn't go to the doctor much, and we were always told it was best to "wait and see." Finally the waiting was over, and it was time to take me to the doctor I hadn't seen in years. It was late in the day and the office was closing. The doctor's unfamiliar face grew serious as he examined me. He explained he needed to put me into the hospital for hydration and testing. A strange mixture of fear and relief flooded into me. There was going to be something else besides the waiting and isolation. I knew my pain saved me and, in a strange way, was to be trusted.

As I entered the hospital I was surprised how my life immediately brightened—the orderly room, the sunshine steaming through the window, the tall nurse with a white cap set on her chestnut hair. I was given a gown with little blue diamonds on it and strings that tied at the waist and neck. My roommate was a girl my age who also had a stomachache. "She has a gallstone," the nurse marveled, as this was the youngest person she had ever known with such a problem. The girl seemed proud of her special stone.

Once a day, the nurse sat on my bed, opened a small bottle of white lotion and rubbed my back. It seemed we could talk about anything we wanted. My developing body with tiny breast buds felt modest and attended to in a way that I had not known possible. Happily, I chatted away. Within days, maybe even hours, my pain lessened into a faint memory. Worried and apprehensive, I wondered where had it gone? Did I still deserve to be here? Had I imagined it, or worse yet, had I lied?

The doctor examined the x-rays of my stomach and discovered an ulcer. He offered no explanation or solution to me. My father sat me down as we packed up my things to leave the hospital.

"We won't tell anyone about this," he decreed.

There was no mention of my parent's fighting, my mother's recurring illness, or my growing confusion. To the doctor and my father, my ulcer was separate from all of this. But I knew. I had learned the power of pain, the importance of listening to the language of the body, and the healing power of touch. None of this could be overshadowed by my father's anger or his denial. The curtain closed. Nothing had changed except that the fighting moved inside me.

The inevitable day came when my mother decided to leave my father. I was twelve and immediately realized that she was leaving me too.

She stopped by the house a week later to pick up some things and to check on the family she'd left behind. It was almost dinnertime and I looked across the kitchen and saw her determined stance at the garage door. I was cooking dinner—something in a big skillet that plugged into the wall. Sizzling, it was liver and onions, unbelievably adult, like I was trying to be.

She came in and began criticizing my father. I shouldn't be cooking dinner, and look how he was creating a Cinderella out of me! And then she left, her words suspended in the air. How could I be a child, how could I stop cooking dinner?

She closed the door and drove away. Her freedom and mine were set apart from one another, and I was left holding the short stick. Stubborn, salty tears fell into that hot skillet. Yet I had something. I had my goodness. I had my honor. I had my love for my mother and her freedom. I believed in her fight and would be loyal to her suffering...to all suffering.

To me, fighting back seemed impossible. Who would I fight? What good would it do? I chose the path of the martyr. I learned to fight with what I thought was my goodness, and pledged my loyalty to the sinking ship. I suffered with an eating disorder in my mid-teens in a desperate attempt to ease my heartbreak over a world I could not control.

This was how in 1968 I came to live alone with my father. Still the main cook in our home, I would read the *Tassajara Bread Book* and the *Moosewood Cookbook* and became fascinated by vegetarian and fresh food cooking. The recipes deviated greatly from our usual diet of pork chops, scalloped potatoes, meatloaf, and peas. One evening, I was inspired to prepare a vegetable omelet for us. I felt creative and empowered as I sautéed vegetables and grated cheese.

Soon my father returned from work, entering the kitchen through the garage door. As I described our menu for the evening, he became agitated and wanted to know what the hell did I think I was doing? I didn't yield, but I didn't provoke. I offered up an explanation of the healthfulness of not always eating meat. His tightly controlled world was unraveling and what was an innocent gesture to me was the last straw for him. He unfurled his anger as he stormed into the living room. Spewing all the toxicity of his life he ranted in profanity and began throwing everything. He turned over tables and ottomans, magazine racks and couches. As a finale, he collapsed in the only standing chair, covered his face, and began to cry. I kneeled beside his chair. I was only fifteen, but I knew it was one of the sanest moments he had ever known. No more pretending, denying, or bullying. His sorrow was finally felt and spoken. For the first time in my life, there was honesty and intimacy between us as the young boy in my father removed his finger from the dike. We righted the furniture and put everything back into the order he revered. Our world reappeared. Together we ate the cold omelet.

That fall I was voted onto the homecoming court as a junior princess at my high school. I had no idea what that meant, and didn't even realize that there had been an election. I was ambivalent about being "popular," and didn't really understand the football scene or how the court would appear on the field during half time. People saw my broad smile, and perhaps my kind heart, but what they couldn't see was that my heart was broken. I felt poorly prepared for the actual event with a mother hospitalized with schizophrenia, a sister away at college, and no fairy godmother to save me. Yet even then, the universe was conspiring to encourage me in some implausible way. My life might have been a complete mess, but somehow that night I became a princess.

I believe I survived my family's suffering by staying present in their chaos and clinging to their craziness like a person capsized at sea. But I knew I needed a different reality. Maybe I couldn't change my family or my genetics, but I did have choices. As young as I was, I could see the futility in the paths that the people around me chose. My sister with her avoidance, my brother with his passive aggression, my father with his cowardly denial, and my mother with her self-preoccupied irresponsibility.

I vowed to learn new skills to prepare me for the inevitable stress of life. I joined a yearlong yoga class offered through the local Unitarian church. I studied consciousness, read books, and sought out friends who thought deeply about life and supported me. I slowly grew stronger, following the echo of my footsteps in our empty house. In some mysterious way, I was being prepared for the ultimate fight.

6.
CARPE DIEM

GREG

AFTER MY FIRST CHEMO TREATMENT, we drove to Oke-mos, the jewel in the ring of suburbs that surrounds Lansing. We were staying with Kate and Mike, our friends of several years. They had always been there for us, and this time was no exception. My cancer was a clarion call for them and they sprang into action. When we returned from the Cancer Center, they rushed to the door and wanted to know what had happened in Ann Arbor.

Mike and I took a short stroll through the maze of intercon-necting streets in their suburb, walking past all the look-alike relatives of their home. I felt weak after the chemo treatment, and I needed to stop frequently. I noticed that there were a lot of houses in the subdivision, but very few people outside. I re-membered late spring nights in my old Grand Rapids; the moist smell of the rain-awakened soil, the sounds of children playing with bikes and balls on the street, mothers telling their children five times to come home—now! Where were the children, the mothers and fathers in Mike's neighborhood? It felt like I was in the middle of a Stephen King novel, and that some scary virus had wiped out all the people. It was desolate.

I realized that something important to me had died. That front porch, front yard culture I knew and loved so much as a child had been replaced by a fenced-in, backyard culture, one in which the properties and the neighbors had been carefully and legally separated.

I felt sad as we took loop after loop through meticulously maintained but empty streets. I knew that the separation between people wasn't just between the houses, it existed within them as well, as family members became seduced by technology. It seemed to me that an unnamed cancer had spread through society while I wasn't looking, destroying the vital cells that were the building blocks of community.

The next morning Kate and Mike came up with a plan. They believed that I was angry about having cancer. Didn't I agree with them that I should get it out? They had just the solution. Kate had several boxes in her garage of assorted dishware that she had either inherited from relatives or grown tired of. Since none of it was of any real value, Kate and Mike suggested that we go into their garage and "have a session together" where I would let my anger out as I smashed the dishes against the brick wall. Didn't I agree that it was a great idea?

Yes, I did, but with one caveat. I would only agree to such a plan if they joined me. Surely they must be angry about something—isn't everybody? There was a thought-filled pause that seemed to last forever. Yes, now that Kate thought about it, there was something she was upset about. Her son's girlfriend had just dumped him to go on to greener pastures, and she was mad at her.

Mike moved the cars out of the garage and into the driveway, and we closed the garage doors to give us a degree of privacy from the neighbors. Like most middle class suburbs, the houses were closely stacked together, separated by thin but important boundaries of shrubs and fences. Kate grabbed two large cardboard boxes from the homemade wooden shelving and opened them. We were ready for action, and I had the honor of throwing the first plate toward the brown brick wall. Here's what the neighbors may or may not have heard that day:

Me (Yelling): You son of a bitch! (Sound of breaking glass)

Kate: I hate you! (Breaking glass)

Me: How could you do this to me? (More glass breaking)

Kate: I hate you!

Me (Screaming now): I'll show you, you little shit!

Kate: (Screaming louder) You're an asshole!

Me (Screaming even louder): You're the real asshole!

On and on it went that dreary spring morning, back and forth, each one of us serving up dishes full of vehemence against the back wall of the garage. The neighbors never called the police to investigate the possibility of domestic violence. If the police had come, I like to think I would have offered them a plate to throw, perhaps even a platter. Surely they too had to be angry about something!

KATHERINE

EVERYTHING CAME TO A STANDSTILL in our lives, including my own attempts to resolve my professional struggle. I was at the end of my rope at work, where I was the proverbial round peg trying to fit into a square hole. Yes, I was a traditionally trained physician, but in my soul I was an eclectic healer. And even more basic, I just wanted time. I wanted more time to understand my patients and empower them to make healthcare decisions that honored the healing potential of their bodies and their lives.

A colleague of mine told me, "You must love your medicine." But truthfully, I didn't love pharmacology or treating symptoms with medications. I could feel my growing reluctance each time I took out my prescription pad. I was passionate, however, about nutrition, herbs, mind-body approaches, insightful conversations, and acupuncture. The fast-paced, drug prescribing way of caring for people left me cold. After twenty years of practice, time was running out. I was not living my truth. And now Greg was ill, throwing into question all my grand plans.

I decided to consult the *I Ching*. Using the *I Ching* had been a practice of mine for the last twenty years or more, and I have grown to trust the insights and wisdom it offers me. Also known as the *Book of Changes*, it is one of the oldest tomes on the planet, and has served countless people as a guide to the way things change. The practice involves forming a question and throwing three coins six times. The coin faces reveal a pattern known as the hexagram. So as Greg watched, I threw the coins. The hexagram first referred to grace, and then it transmuted into community. It described how my personal success would serve as an example and benefit others, as well as myself. The hexagram also contained this warning: *Are your goals consonant with the wellbeing of those dear to you? This is not the time to strike out as an individual.*

Even though I knew what I needed to do, I saw the risk to my family. My path was so linked to Greg, that I couldn't imagine going forward as he retreated. Could I launch this project of a lifetime without him? I knew the answer. I needed and depended on his love and commitment in all our major endeavors. As I contemplated the bank loans and real estate, I became dizzy and distracted. I knew in my heart that his health needed to take priority over everything else. Again, I would have to wait to make a change, not from doubts, but because of love.

GREG

CANCER SUDDENLY CHANGED THE RULES of the game and now I was playing for keeps and with a new intensity. My eyes began to tear as I watched Emerson's blond hair blow freely in the wind as we drove home to Traverse City. I was especially grateful that she remained protected by her childhood innocence and had no idea what I was going through. Being sick to her meant having a boo-boo; something that hurt, but something Mommy and Daddy could fix easily with a Dora the Explorer band-aid and a special kiss.

It was no big deal for her to be left with our caring friends when Katherine and I went off to the Cancer Center, and I wanted to keep it that way as long as possible. My suffering remained invisible to her young eyes. There would be so many things in the future that we would have to explain. *Why doesn't Dad-da have any hair? Dad-da not hungry? Dad-da sick? Where is Dad-da?* (crying) *I want my Dad-da!* (screaming).

How would I ever be able explain cancer to her? It was a strange and violent sickness that even Katherine and I didn't fully understand. I was sure that at some point during my treatment a social worker would give us a book that would help us explain the whole thing to her and "prepare" her for my death. The book would probably be some sort of picture book with an older animal, a grandfather, or maybe even a father, sick in bed while little animal doctors and nurses attended to him.

How could we tell a three-year-old who was at the start of her life that I was going to die? She was just beginning to get to know me! There were so many things I was looking forward to doing with her! I wanted to take her to music lessons, watch her play sports, everything! Pretty soon she wouldn't have a father, she wouldn't even have a clear memory of ever having one! Would this cripple her psychologically? Would she be doomed by a fatal attraction to older men, unconsciously trying to seek the lost love of a father figure?

And how was I supposed to explain to Emerson where people go after they die when I had no idea myself?

I had spent much of my life pondering the question of life after death. I was fairly certain that even if there was a heaven, it was not going to be the heaven of my Catholic childhood, the one where Saint Peter, the celestial concierge, checked you in to a luxurious hotel that would make the Ritz-Carlton look like Motel 6. If that were the case, I was in major trouble. I was certain I didn't have enough reward points to qualify for a room.

I didn't believe in purgatory at all, much less in hell. Purgatory is such a bizarre concept; a place where you basically rotated on a rotisserie and were tortured over white-hot coals while you worked off your sins. Oddly enough, that was just like what going to church felt like to me as a youngster, squirming on the rock-hard pew, waiting for mass to end.

I read many books, some by philosophers, some by theologians, and some by spiritual teachers. I also attended retreats, went to different churches, attended a synagogue, had my palm read—all in my attempt to search for the meaning of life. In the end what resonated most was the work of Dostoyevsky, the great Russian novelist. I was absolutely fascinated with the account of his arrest and subsequent mock execution when his life was spared at the very last second. The characters in his novels moved me to tears; they were people I could identify with, people struggling to understand how the innocent could suffer. They were people searching for God.

My favorite novel of Dostoyevsky's—for that matter my favorite book of all time—is *The Brothers Karamazov*. Here, in one book, Dostoyevsky reveals to the reader the entire canvas: life, death, good, evil, family, conflict, God, and Satan. I was especially taken by the life story of the elder Zosima, whose older brother has a life changing epiphany on his deathbed. His brother wakes up in the very last minute from a lifetime of self-absorbed complacency and grasps the miracle of life. His brother's realization is so powerful that it changes Zosima from an arrogant, narcissistic, military man into a monk deeply connected to the miracle of life.

I could relate to the story in so many ways. Where had I been all of these years? True, I had accomplished a great many things: I had earned several degrees, taught numerous students, helped scores of clients, had good friends, married a wonderful woman, fathered a miracle child. But I never really "got it." I took everything for granted, assuming it would all be there tomorrow, and the day after that, and the day after that.

It was Dostoyevsky who showed me the way to my own epiphany. Life was a miracle, a gift, and it was short—Carpe Diem! Even before cancer, I enthusiastically shared what I discovered with my patients and lectured to community groups about it.

I "got" the fact that my life, like everything else, was impermanent. I understood it intellectually, but, like most people, it wasn't until I was diagnosed with cancer that I felt it.

The fact of the matter was that the show was coming to an end, now, not 30 years from now. I would be lucky to smell the spring flowers one more time, to hear the cheerful song of my favorite bird, the cardinal, and to see the crabapple tree in our backyard get all gussied up in her deep pink blossom dress.

Emerson and I stuck our hands out of the Subaru's windows and laughed together as the wind pushed our palms up and away. I knew it wouldn't be long before the day would come when she would find this boring and want to go on to the next thing. Would she be lucky enough to rediscover the joy of hand surfing when she became a parent?

I couldn't handle the painful realization that I would not be around for the big things in her life: kindergarten, swimming lessons, and teaching her how to ride a bike. I wanted to be the one who took her to the mall parking lot on a Sunday morning to teach her how to drive. Even though I would probably cry my eyes out, I wanted to be there when we said our first real goodbyes as we dropped her off at a too-far-away university. I couldn't accept the thought that I'd miss it all. I had to find some way to live!

7.

THE CHEMO KNITTING GROUP

GREG

WHEN WE RETURNED HOME TO TRAVERSE CITY on April 12th, we were surprised to find three-foot long stems of tiny white flowers hanging like clusters of grapes from our six-foot cane plant—the plant had never bloomed during the three years it had been in the bedroom!

Suddenly, I became overwhelmed by a strange sensation. I could actually smell the fragrant flowers! I closed off my right nostril with my index finger and tried to inhale through the left nostril alone. Air moist with humidity poured through my nasal passage. I could breathe through my left nostril for the first time in six months! Could it be? Was the tumor…gone?

It all felt so strange. What was even more bizarre was my immediate feeling that the rare blossoms were a message sent to us from our dear friend Marilyn. Only she would know how desperate we were for a sign of hope. If anybody could send a message from the other side, it would be her.

We returned to the Cancer Center a week later, fueled by our hopes that my tumor was receding, that I was killing it, that we were going to win the fight after all. As we navigated crowded hallways, I caught a glimpse of my chemo doctor, Dr. Francisco, surrounded by a circle of attentive residents.

"Dr. Francisco," I shouted, unable to contain my excitement, "I'm getting better! I can breathe again!"

"What?" He seemed irritated at the interruption.

"I said I'm getting better…I can breathe! Through my nostril! I smelled some flowers!" I exclaimed.

He shifted his full focus on me and slowly registered who I was. "Well," he said, dismissively, "I need some clinical evidence." He abruptly turned on his heels and began to walk down the hall, followed by an obedient cadre of residents.

I was furious. I couldn't believe how he had treated me! My anger chased him down the hall. "I am getting better!" I shouted. "I'm going to come back here in five years and show you! You're going to write about me!"

Katherine grabbed my arm in an effort to restrain me and hustled me back through the clinic. She was everything I ever needed in my life—best friend, lover, true healer—and now she became my trainer, my handler, the Angelo Dundee to my Ali. I reluctantly agreed with her that I needed to fight my cancer, not my doctors.

Later that day, I had my official appointment with Dr. Francisco. There was no acknowledgement of our confrontation in the hallway. We discussed continuing the chemotherapy treatments in Traverse City while we waited to return to Ann Arbor for the radiation. He remained unmoved by my ability to breathe again through my left nostril. His opinion was that "perhaps" the chemotherapy had "temporarily slowed down the progression" of the cancer. He offered no encouragement, no hope. Deflated but not defeated, we left for home.

TRAVERSE CITY IS A QUINTESSENTIAL SMALL TOWN where people seem to know what happens to you before you do. Two weeks after my diagnosis, many people were aware of the fact that I had cancer. By the time we returned from my appointment with Dr. Francisco, Katherine and I had received an abundance of cards from people wishing me well. Several mentioned that they had been praying for me, and one family arranged to have a special prayer service said at their church. We also received a card from a Native American tribe somewhere out West, informing us that an anonymous person had told them about my plight, and that they were holding a healing ceremony for me.

One of the hardest things was telling my patients that I was closing my practice. The cold, hard facts of the matter were that I was scheduled to go back to the Cancer Center for two solid months of additional chemo, as well as daily doses of radiation. I knew I would become very sick. Even if I did make it back home I would be in no shape to work. Still, I felt terrible about leaving my patients, especially since several of them had already been abandoned once before in their lives.

I decided to write them a letter, which would probably confirm their worst fears. Yet first and foremost I needed to tell them the truth, just as I had encouraged them to do. The letter went like this:

Dear Friends,

I am writing you to inform you that I have recently been diagnosed with cancer. As such, I will be in Ann Arbor for an extended stay to receive the necessary treatment, and I will need to focus all of my energy on healing. I have made the difficult but necessary decision to temporarily close my office.

Even though I won't be able to see you during this time, you will be with me in my memory and in my heart. I'll be thinking about you as you face your challenges, and I continue to wish you the best in those endeavors.

*I realize that this news may be quite difficult for you, and
I am sorry that I won't be able to see you at this time. If you
would like to transfer to another psychologist, please let me
know, and I will do my best to help arrange this.*

*If you would like updates on my progress, please send
me your email, and I will send a group email when I know
more.*

What I didn't say was precisely what I wasn't ready to concede:
that that I was dying and would likely never see any of them again.
I wasn't ready to call it a game. I felt that my job here on Earth was
far from finished.

I'VE MET SEVERAL ONCOLOGISTS IN MY LIFE, and there's
not a single one who I'd describe as having an ebullient personality.
It may seem ironic, but I've met undertakers with more life in them.
Now it was time for me to meet the Traverse City oncologist who
would supervise the administration of my chemotherapy while I
waited ten days to return to Ann Arbor to begin my radiation.

Dr. Bixby did little, if anything, to challenge my stereotype of oncologists. He was kind of kind, and by that I mean he was quick to
see me at Katherine's request. Just like the doctors before him, he
seemed interested in what I had, though not so much in who I was
or how I felt. I thought about the days when I would go on morning
rounds with the resident physicians and listen to them talk about
their patients: "He's the heart attack in 3308." or "Let's go see the
stroke downstairs." I knew the doctors in Ann Arbor saw me as the
"rare tumor" or "SNUC."

Dr. Bixby had never seen a patient with my type of cancer before,
and was more than happy to go with the treatment protocol dictat-

ed by Dr. Francisco. He rubber-stamped the orders for the chemo and I went down the hallway to face my lifelong nemesis, the IV.

Like bars, no two chemo lounges are alike. Each one has a personality all its own. The chemo lounge at the hospital in Ann Arbor was enormous, with a couple dozen recliner chairs arranged in a semicircle around a long, island-like structure that served as the nurses' workspace. The chemo was housed in a separate storage area and was replenished as needed by the pharmacy technicians.

Dr. Bixby's chemo lounge, by comparison, was a much smaller and more intimate space. Four recliners faced one another in a small circle, like a group of knitters might form as they gathered together to make Christmas presents for grandchildren. There was no opportunity for any hanky-panky this time around. I had proven at the Cancer Center that I could survive the injection of Etopside and cisplatin without having a heart attack, and from now on I would receive my treatment out in the open with everyone else.

Cyndi, my nurse, sat me down in a recliner. I knew what was coming, and a chill crept over my entire body in anticipation.

"My, you're cold!" Cyndi exclaimed. She fetched a green itchy blanket to tuck around me.

I confessed my fear of needles straightaway, and she assured me that, "We would take our time," and that she would do everything she could to make me feel comfortable. I never did warm up to the idea of the IV. Cyndi extended my right arm and pressed her thumb against my forearm in an attempt to find a "good one." Finally she found a decent vein, swabbed it with alcohol, and inserted the needle. A sharp pain shot through my body, and my eyes rolled back into my head

There was a long pause, followed by the words you never ever want to hear from a doctor or nurse. "Oh, oh!" Cyndi said with a slight air of exasperation. The painfully placed IV wasn't working, as my blood was not flowing up the plastic tube. She was truly sorry—maybe we should try my left arm instead? She assured me that what happened wasn't that unusual. Some people's veins were "just like that," and were easier to get at on one side than the other.

Once the IV was truly in, I sat back in the recliner and joined in the conversation with the other people receiving their respective cocktails. No one mentioned what kind of cancer he or she had. I don't think that the word "cancer" was uttered even once. Instead we talked about life—real life. There were funny stories about the hi-jinks of grandchildren, excitement about what this year's garden might produce, and overly optimistic predictions about the Detroit Tigers baseball season. Our little chemo-knitting group took each of these stories and stitched them together, creating a rich tapestry of our lives.

Nobody in the group talked about what incredible thing they had done, what company they may have started. Not a soul peeped about who they knew or what famous person they might have met. Cancer and the looming specter of death stripped away the veneer of pretense and revealed our true nature—that we were in fact equals—no better, no worse than the person in the next chair. The truth that I learned that day was simple, yet profound; we were much more alike than we were different.

WE BEGAN TO PREPARE FOR OUR TRIP downstate to the Cancer Center. My treatment would last eight weeks, with daily radiation treatments interspersed with a few more rounds of chemotherapy. But where would we live? The four-hour commute each way was tiresome and entirely out of the question.

The best option was to "couch-surf" with various friends in the Lansing area. It would still be an hour commute each way, but it was much more doable than the four-hour drive from our house to Ann Arbor. Our friends were eager to pitch in and help in any way possible, and we were convinced that we could work out a week-by-week schedule between them.

The idea of staying with friends definitely felt better than staying at a motel or the Ronald McDonald House, yet there was something about it that didn't feel quite right. I was already having side effects from the chemo and starting to feel sick. I was exhausted, and I had lost my sense of taste. I knew that any day now I would start to lose my hair. There was little question that our friends would take on the responsibility of caring for us with great love and compassion, but I wanted to be neither a burden or a reminder of their own mortality.

The thought of asking my friends to disrupt their lives to care for me was just too much. I had discovered through many years of experience visiting friends and relatives that Ben Franklin had been right when he said that fish and visitors stink after three days. What about a visitor who stayed for a week while he was dying before your eyes?

Then, I received a call from Sue, a former patient of mine. She didn't call me because she needed my help again; she was calling to offer me help. Why didn't Katherine and I stay at their family cottage on Silver Lake? They weren't going to need it until July, and it would be perfect for us as it was only 20 minutes away from the Cancer Center. She wouldn't listen to my objections and all but demanded we accept.

Initially I felt awkward about Sue's more than generous offer. It had been drilled into me during training that it was important to have strict "boundaries" between yourself and your patients. I was taught to view patients who offered any kind of gift with a degree of psychoanalytic suspicion. There was always a dark motivation lurking somewhere behind the gift that needed to be brought into the daylight by the brilliant interpretations of the analyst.

All in all, though, I didn't agree with a lot of what I heard in graduate school. I was as skeptical of the belief that there was only one way to be a psychotherapist, as I was that there was only one way to believe in God. I never could buy into the idea that there was always something wrong with a client who wanted to do something nice for you. Didn't Freud say, "Sometimes a cigar is only a cigar"? I never expected someone to bring a cup of coffee to share with me during his or her session, but I would always accept it. Not only did I accept it, but I would also express my gratitude. Why spoil someone's effort to do something nice for you with an interpretation that had more to do with your unconscious than theirs?

That may not have been what an East Coast psychoanalyst would do, but the only thing I wanted to be was me. If I couldn't muster the courage to be me, regardless of what others thought, then how could I honestly encourage my clients to be who they really were?

Sue promised the lakefront cottage would be comfortable, and had a layered deck for relaxing. In the spirit of full disclosure, she added one caveat: The neighbors behind her cottage were "a little different." Luke, the father of the clan, had done time in prison for either selling drugs or committing child abuse. She was quick to add that even though her family had never had any problems with them, she wanted us to be aware, especially since we would have little Emerson with us.

Even with the suspicious neighbors, Katherine and I agreed that staying at Sue's cottage sounded like a good idea. The account of the neighbors was disturbing, but we figured Sue would not have offered her cottage if she truly believed we would be endangered. Of course, we would lock doors at night and keep a close eye on Emerson.

8.

SILVER LAKE

GREG

AFTER STUFFING THE SUBARU TO THE BRIM, we scooped up Emerson and backed out of our driveway. My heart was heavy as I watched our home disappear in the rearview mirror. Leaving had such a disturbing feeling of finality to it. The odds were that I would return either dead in the back of a hearse, or on the edge of life from the chemo and intense radiation.

We found the cottage on a dirt road among a row of similar cottages that faced south across Silver Lake, one of several minuscule lakes that dotted the forested countryside west of Ann Arbor.

Sue's cottage had a nicely kept, bright green yard between it and the dirt road. The nefarious neighbor lived in the dark shadow of Sue's cottage, across the dirt access road. Luke's driveway was crammed with several vehicles in various states of disrepair. The smallish home hadn't seen a hammer or a fresh coat of paint in ages, and the yard was strewn with orphaned bikes and toys. I wondered what really went on inside the house, but quickly realized I didn't want to know.

Sue's two-story cottage was as clean and nicely appointed as we had imagined. The first floor featured a generous kitchen, bath, and living room with a sliding glass door that accessed the deck and lake, while the sleeping areas were upstairs. I flopped down on the leather couch and looked out over the lake. There was not a drop of gas left in my tank. I felt bad about not being able to help Katherine unpack the car, watch Emerson, and set up base camp. The cancer was taking its toll, cell by cell.

We awoke the next morning as rays of a magnificent sunrise filtered through the bedroom curtains. It had been a fitful night for me as I went over and over my usual laundry list of worries: cancer, chemo, IV's, radiation, death, Katherine and Emerson's life left in ruins. Round and round the merry-go-round of my mind spun, and at the end of the ride the only thing I had to show for it was feeling even more depleted than the day before. Worry is one of the worst addictions ever; even though you realize it's stealing your life away, you can't seem to do a thing to stop it.

KATHERINE

THE COTTAGE OPENED ITS ARMS to us and we stepped into its unfamiliar embrace on the Saturday before Mother's Day. We arrived at sunset, and Emerson, thinking we were on vacation, insisted on putting on her bathing suit and red flowered sunhat. The lake water had just thawed from the winter freeze and was icy cold. Emerson didn't mind and squealed as she dangled her toes over the edge of the dock.

Kate, our dish-throwing friend, had packed a supper of pasta and salad to help with the first steps of the journey. Despite the coolness of the late afternoon, we decided to eat outside. We lingered on the deck as the sun set and took in the details of our surroundings. An oriole serenaded us from the sycamore tree and we marveled at its brilliant orange color in the long rays of light. Greg reminded Emerson, again and again, to close the screen door as she ran in and out of our new home.

On my birthday, the week before, Greg had given me a journal. I cried when I unwrapped it and pressed the blank pages with their foreboding emptiness to my chest. I knew one day they would be filled with what lay ahead. Now with trepidation, sadness, and uncertainty I opened it and uncapped my pen. The early spring mist lingered over the silky silver water, and I took my first deep breath in weeks.

After just one month, the cancer had affected us deeply. Seriousness hung over every moment, and the perspective was humbling. We looked more deeply into each other's eyes and listened even more carefully when the other spoke. A strange blend of politeness and gentleness guided our interactions. Death was on our shoulder, and our appreciation for what we had, and what might soon be gone, intensified.

As sobering as this was, life in all its magical radiance sat squarely upon the other shoulder. We were amazed at how quickly Greg's treatment started, at the outpouring of love from family and friends, and the blessing of our living arrangements just outside Ann Arbor. Throughout it all, we chose our attitude of love for it was the only freedom we truly had.

MY DREAMS BECAME MORE TRANSPARENT AND IMPORTANT. I wrote them down, like inner road maps, next to reflections on our daily trials. The first night in the cottage I dreamt of a spider weaving a complex web. All the threads of the web rolled into a ball, and then the unseen spider pulled at the delicate filament and it took form. A huge shimmering web appeared with the tiniest of seeds suspended in it. I watched it like some kaleidoscopic miracle, a Milky Way, and then I flew through it with another person. People gathered below, and just as we turned to look at one another, we began to fall.

I began to stir and surface. I wanted to return to the dream and fly on into the night but I was awake. As I opened the journal and my hand met the page, I knew I was being guided to connect with spirit and practice transcendence. I wondered if the seeds in the web were related to Greg's cancer. Had they been caught in the delicate knowing of the universe?

As we wrote together in the morning silence, Greg's family was making their several-hour drive from Grand Rapids to celebrate Mother's Day with us—our first time together since the fall. I savored the chance to do something "normal." Yet once the bustle of their arrival settled into catching up on each other's busy lives, I felt odd. It was difficult for me to relate to the digital photographs of our nephew's prom with the fancy dresses and limos. The pork roast and potato salad left me feeling empty. I was totally out of step when we began the family ritual of card playing, usually a raucous, boisterous affair.

I wanted to talk about Greg, discover what needed to be said, and respond to questions that needed to be understood. No tears were shed, and few questions were asked. Were they too afraid to talk, or was it politeness? They didn't seem to know what to say, so they said nothing.

GREG

MOTHER'S DAY WAS THE FIRST TIME my parents and I were able to get together since I was diagnosed, and I wondered if it would be the last. My parents and three sisters had been shocked by the news. I'd called my parents soon after we had received the diagnosis.

"Hay-lo," my dad answered in his signature fashion.

"Dad...I...uh," I sputtered, tears running down my cheek into the mouthpiece of the black phone. "Dad, I . . .um . . ."

"Yes," he replied with an impatient tone, trying to prime my pump.

"I need…to talk to you…and Mom. Is she there?"

"Mary!" he shouted. No luck. "Mary! It's Greg!"

I could hear my mother's response in the distance, "What?"

"It's Greg! He's on the phone! He wants to talk with you!"

"I'm coming, I'm coming! You don't have to shout!"

I hesitated to tell my parents how I really felt; I had never felt safe revealing what dreams fueled my passions or the dark nightmares that chased me at night. That all changed the night I called to tell them I had cancer. Cancer had forced my hand, and I could no longer continue to pretend that everything was okay. I blurted out the truth into the cordless phone—I was sick with a rare, bad cancer, and I was going to die very soon. I lost control of my emotions and sobbed like their baby that I once was. My dam of inhibition collapsed, and everything came flooding out, wave after wave that night—how I didn't want to die, how I didn't want to leave Katherine, how it would affect Emerson.

The combination of unexpected news and my onslaught of emotions overwhelmed them. They didn't know what to say. I can't remember either of my parents ever discussing their feelings. I was sure they were in there somewhere, but my folks were private people whose primary mission in life was to never burden their children. I wasn't looking for a whole lot that night; I stopped doing that a long time ago. They were my parents, and I simply wanted them to know.

Five weeks later, as we ate our holiday meal of pork roast and salad, Mother's Day felt like a cross between a graduation party and a memorial service. There wasn't a peep out of anyone about how scared they might be, and nobody wanted to hear the grisly details of the treatments that were ahead of me.

We said goodbye to my family and thanked them for coming as they climbed into the white minivan for their trip home. I felt so bad for my parents as they struggled to get into the car. I had watched them, for what seemed like forever, battling through one illness or another, decade after decade. I had anticipated losing them for such a long time; it had never occurred to me that I might beat them to the finish line.

KATHERINE

SEAN, GREG'S YOUNGEST NEPHEW, WAS RELUCTANT to go. He looked at Greg with fondness and his lower lip trembled, yet words eluded him. What could he possibly say? Greg's father fumbled with the car keys and stood in the driveway with the car door open. I could see the pain in his eyes. The car drove off, and the dust settled on the dirt road. Within minutes, out of nowhere, an unexpected afternoon storm broke loose. Dark clouds eclipsed the afternoon sun, and lightning, thunder, and torrential rain passed over the cottage. Emerson awoke crying from her nap. My pager began to beep at random intervals for unknown reasons. The thunder rumbled for hours.

GREG

AS THE SUN PEEKED OUT after the afternoon storm I looked across the road toward the neighbor's house and saw a slightly built man trying to resuscitate one of the half-dead cars in the driveway. I had an intuition that I should reach out to him and let him know we weren't there looking for any kind of trouble.

As I walked up the dirt drive I could hear cuss words flying out like sparks from under the hood of a beat-up Ford van. "Luke?" I ventured.

"Whaddya want?" a muffled voice replied from under the hood.

"I'm your new neighbor, Greg. I just wanted to introduce myself and let you know that I'll be staying at Sue's cottage for the next few weeks."

"All righty," the voice replied as the man slowly uncoiled himself and turned to face me. His reddish brown hair was disheveled, and his hands and grimy V-neck T-shirt were covered with grease. I was surprised when he met my smile with a smile of his own. He didn't seem bothered about being interrupted. "Whatchya say you were gonna do again?" he asked.

"I just thought I'd come over and introduce myself," I replied. "My family will be staying over at Sue's for the next couple of months while I go back and forth to the hospital for cancer treatment."

Luke wanted to know what kind of cancer I had, so I gave him the *Reader's Digest* abridged version. He seemed genuinely concerned. He surprised me when he wanted to know if he could do anything for me while I was at the lake. I didn't have the feeling I was talking to some monster that was out to get me. I was already facing a real monster, and one that was eating me alive.

EARLY THE NEXT DAY I went to the Cancer Center to have my follow up CT Scan. It had been ordered by the doctors after my second round of chemotherapy and would be critical to them in designing the radiation program for the next eight weeks.

The radiation area was separate from the rest of the Cancer Center, with a parking area and entrance of its own. The waiting area was a semicircular room with a tall ceiling, several large windows, and a curved desk for the kind receptionist who greeted me with forms to fill out. On the wall opposite were two huge, metal doors. I was afraid of what went on behind them, although I knew I was about to find out. I peeked up from the two-year-old *Sports Illustrated* I was pretending to read, and watched the doors open and close like the jaws of a dragon, devouring patients one by one.

The hungry doors swung open, and a muscular black man emerged holding a green chart. "Dr. Holmes...Dr. Holmes?" he called out. I was so scared that I hesitated for a second to fess up and claim my identity. Finally I gave in and weakly raised my hand, getting it up about as high as my shoulder.

"Dr. Holmes! Why there you are! Good morning to you, sir! Lee-on here!" he said by way of introduction. I looked up at the large figure that towered over me; the distance between our physical statures and moods couldn't have been greater. The muscles that protruded from the short sleeves of his dark blue medical scrubs were like the Rocky Mountains compared to the flatlands of my biceps. His enormous white smile was as wide as the Mississippi, whereas my own smile had disappeared long ago like a dried-up water hole in the arid desert.

"Lee-on's gonna show you around just a little bit, take you downstairs!" Leon's speech was as big and as bold as his body. It was full of exclamations, and short on the little things like personal pronouns. I wondered what he thought about me and my sick, little white body.

When Leon pushed a button and the doors opened, I thought of the inscription above the door to Hell in Dante's *Inferno*: "Abandon hope all ye who enter here." Although I'd summoned the courage to go into the heart of the radiation center, I refused to abandon hope. Like Pandora before me, hope was all that was left.

There was a nursing station inside the double doors, surrounded by several examination rooms. Leon helped me climb up on a gurney and tightened a couple of straps around me. "Are you ready?" he asked. "Lee-on's gonna give you a little ride! Here we go!" And off we did go, racing down the halls as if he was taking me to the emergency room. Leon was the kind of person who has only one speed—faster than fast. We took the elevator down to the basement level, and Leon pushed my gurney at a rapid clip through a dark, tunnel-like structure, finally coming to rest at the clinic where the CT scan machine was located.

Leon grabbed the chart that had somehow managed to stay balanced on my chest during our wild ride. "We're gonna have this CT done in record time!" he announced, and based on my experience so far, I believed him. "Now Leon's gonna have to give you a little poke!" he said as he grabbed my arm and placed it on a small stand by the gurney. I tried to tell Leon about the difficulties that the infusion nurse experienced starting my IV, but he interrupted. "That's because Lee-on didn't do it!" he explained as he kept on moving.

That morning I discovered that humans could levitate. My entire body left the gurney when Leon missed my vein and hit a nerve instead. The pain was so intense that I thought I was going to die right there in the CT clinic. What was really scary was Leon's refusal to acknowledge my pain and his mistake. The miss only added fuel to the fire of his intensity. "Lee-on's gonna get it this time!" he exclaimed. I closed my eyes as tight as I could and prayed he was right. By luck or design the second needle found its way into my vein.

After the scan was over and Leon had pulled the IV out of my battered arm, he pushed the gurney back down the hall and we rode up the elevator in silence. I hoped Leon had pushed the right buttons on the control panel when he did the CT. He had certainly pushed the wrong buttons in me.

9.

THE GREEN MASK

GREG

EARLY THE NEXT MORNING, Katherine and I drove from Sue's cottage to the radiation center. It was difficult to focus, as I was hung over from the Klonopin that I had taken the night before. I was beginning to develop a psychological dependency on the sedative, yet I was so anxious that I couldn't sleep without it. Becoming an addict was the least of my concerns. I would deal with that problem later on—if there was a later on. Getting rest was of utmost concern, and if I had to knock myself out to get some sleep, well that was the way it was.

I was amazed by the unfailingly upbeat moods of the receptionists and the nurses at the radiation center. How could they be so pleasant and cheerful after everything they saw? Day after day they witnessed people of all ages become sick from the powerful radiation and wither up like prunes. Sometimes the patients would disappear completely. The buoyant attitudes and big smiles of the staff stood in stark contrast to the etched-in-stone faces of the oncologists. I hoped the doctors were different people when they went home. I doubted it.

A nurse escorted Katherine and me through the two swinging doors, past the nurses' station, and into a small exam room. The examination rooms in all of my oncologists' offices were virtually indistinguishable from one another. They were small interior spaces without windows, fresh air or plants, each artificially lit by too-bright fluorescent ceiling lights. There was no artwork—not even cheap travel posters—on any of the walls of the tiny square boxes. The only color was the steel gray of the cabinetry. There were no cute pictures of family members on the sterilized countertops. There was not a single sign of life.

I plunked myself down on the exam chair that sat in the middle of the room. Katherine pulled a chair up beside me and grabbed my hand for dear life.

KATHERINE

IT WAS UNFATHOMABLE TO ME that there would be another side to this—that in eight weeks the treatment would be over. The future stood before me like a formidable mountain and I could not imagine how we'd reach the other side. I was literally locked in the moment-by-moment unfolding of the experience. For years I had studied mindfulness, and countless times encouraged myself to remain in the moment, this very one, and not ricochet into the past or the future. Now all I could see was this day and its poignancy. I realized that my mind, so used to being in control, needed to take its hands off the steering wheel and surrender. I had to trust that in surrendering we would find our power.

Greg was ecstatic that he could breathe through his left nostril and that his sense of smell was back. When he spoke, his voice was clear and no longer sounded like he had a permanent cold. But sitting in the waiting room, preparing for Greg's name to be called, my Zen mind dissolved into a million questions. He had completed the first two rounds of chemotherapy and was about to begin the eight weeks of radiation. Had the tumor responded to chemotherapy? What did the most recent CT scan say? How did the doctor know how much radiation Greg needed? Did it matter that he had never smoked or that he was so "healthy"? When would we say "enough" and get him a feeding tube? I was consumed with worry that the treatments had the power to destroy him.

I quieted my mind and looked at Greg's face. I was here for him, and in this moment, there was nothing else to do. I looked around the waiting room. In the corner was a children's play area with a basket of well-used toys. A young girl kneeled at the basket and her small hands stroked Big Bird's balding head. I thought of all the children who had come before us, and knew that one day Emerson would play here too.

Greg's name was called and broke through my daydream. The nurse led us through a maze of hallways to a small exam room. Minutes passed as we collected our thoughts and braced ourselves for the encounter that would set everything in motion. Dr. Abdul bustled in. He was short in both stature and words. He spoke with an unfamiliar Middle Eastern accent that I couldn't quite place. After a formal greeting and introductions, he placed a copy of Greg's CT scan on an illuminated surface so that we could all see its prophetic images. I realized that this was the first time anyone had actually sat with us and looked at Greg's films. No one had taken the time, or perhaps had the courage, to do so. My mouth went dry and I blinked away my tears.

We circled around the images as if they were military maps, planning our strategy to confront the enemy. Our fragile optimism was dashed when he announced that he did not see the improvement Greg and I had expected with his newfound power to smell. He pointed to the tumor and drew a dramatic red arrow to emphasize its proximity to Greg's left eye. The circles he drew in different colored wax pencils accentuated how the cancer had invaded bone tissue and was slowly taking over the delicate passages of Greg's sinuses.

GREG

THERE WAS A RAPID-FIRE SERIES of five knocks on the exam room door, and before we could say, "Come in," Dr. Abdul burst into the room. He was one of the head honchos in the radiation oncology department at the university, and it was clear we were in the presence of a man on a mission.

Dr. Abdul pulled out several images of my CT scan from an over-sized sleeve. The black and white images looked ghostly to me. The only thing I could make out was the general contour of my head and neck. Dr. Abdul quickly traced the scans as he described the size and location of the tumor in his businesslike manner. He explained that the tumor was eroding the bone that separated my sinus cavity from my brain. I wondered, terrified, how long it would take for the tumor to break through that firewall and begin eating my brain. As I watched Dr. Abdul's finger trace the scan, I understood why the nervous neurosurgeon had refused to meet with us.

Dr. Abdul squirted some anesthetic medication up my nostril and stuck a lengthy endoscope up my nose and into my sinus area to get a look-see at the deadly tumor. I didn't understand why he needed to look at it since he had pictures of the dang thing right in his hand, but I kept my mouth shut. Even though I was anesthetized, it felt weird to have the tube twisting around inside my head.

He briefly went over the possible side effects of the radiation. There was an 80 percent chance that the radiation would destroy the optic nerve and, therefore, the vision in my left eye. There would likely be damage to my salivary glands, and the reduction of sal-ivation would lead to problems with my teeth. My thyroid gland would be toast, and there would be the usual issues with fatigue, weight loss, and change of appetite. Ironically, the radiation itself was carcinogenic—the treatment could trigger yet another cancer in the future! He mentioned that I might become depressed, but he didn't seem to notice my mood was already in the toilet.

Dr. Abdul concluded the appointment by informing us that radiation treatment would begin the next afternoon. He asked if I still wanted to proceed, and I replied quietly that I did. I signed the requisite forms and that was that. The sessions would last approximately 30 to 45 minutes each day, five days a week for eight weeks. Our visit ended, and off went Dr. Abdul with his resident. I could hear five quick knocks on the door of the room next to me.

KATHERINE

I WONDERED HOW ALL OF THIS COULD BE TRUE. If I didn't know better, I would never concede that anything was wrong with him—he looked like a man in perfect health.

My eyes returned to the black and white images on the screen and I heard the seriousness in Dr. Adbul's voice. He admitted his own uncertainty about how much radiation was necessary and revealed the slippery slope of the proper dose. Too little, and the cancer cells would survive. Too much, and it would destroy Greg's left eye.

Over the next several days a group of physicists would develop the program for the conformal radiation that would target the radiation beams to hit Greg's tumor from multiple angles. The degree of precision and intensity was both reassuring and shocking. Dr. Abdul agreed to reevaluate the plan in five weeks after Greg's next CT scan. At that time he would decide whether he could lessen the intensity of the radiation.

It took time for everything to sink in. When we entered the cottage, Greg began to cry. His preoccupation with the logistics of leaving home and coming to the cottage had distracted him from his feelings. Now, the treatment schedule was set and ready to begin. I was sad, yet relieved to see his tears; there was honesty in them.

He called several of his good friends and talked to them. They were eager to hear his voice and offer their encouragement.

Emerson and I played on the back stoop. We perched there, listening to Greg's distant voice amidst the smells of the lilac bush. Finally, he put the phone down on the kitchen table and stepped out into the fading afternoon light. Restless, we set off together down the unfamiliar dirt road that circled the lake. Emerson's short legs set our pace. Strolling along, we imagined the lives of the unseen people in the tidy cottages. It was a weekday in late spring and many homes were still closed up, but their essence remained—some with well-tended gardens and knickknacks, others shuttered, with flaking paint and brown grass yards.

Even now Greg was such a wonderful companion. He teased us into laughter and helped us feel connected to the world, to this new place, and to our old friends. He was doing everything to stay present with us as the sharks circled beneath him. That night as I walked beside him with my hand in his, the dust barely stirred under his sandals. It broke my heart open that even now he made it all look easy.

GREG

I WAS DISTRAUGHT with the news that I would likely lose my vision and thought about nothing else that day. We made our way through the small, gentrified town of Dexter, and headed toward Sue's cottage on Silver Lake. I knew I would lose my depth perception when I couldn't see out of both eyes, but what else would happen? Would they remove the dead eye and replace it with a glass eye, or would I be forced to wear a thin black patch over it like a pirate? What if I injured my other eye and lost my vision altogether?

Would my brain be the next thing to go? Was this how it was going to be—I would die piece by piece?

I was so relieved when we finally pulled in the driveway of the cottage and I saw Emerson. She ran headfirst through the cottage and launched herself into my eager arms. She was my polar opposite, a person full of vim and vigor, someone just starting her life journey. She loved spending time with our friend Kate, but now was eager to be with me. Emerson was a physical child who loved it when I got down on all fours to play horsey around the back forty of the living room.

I looked carefully at her big blue eyes. I wanted to be sure that I saw everything—everything—before I went blind. Much of my life had been one big blur as I raced down the expressway of life, trying to get from here to there to the next thing, etc., etc. What had I really seen? When all was said and done, where had I really been? I knew that it was impossible to stop and smell every flower, but couldn't I have just slowed down, once in a while, and driven the speed limit? And why had I wasted so much time worrying about hundreds and hundreds of things that never happened?

One night, several years ago, Katherine and I were driving downstate for a visit. We were flying down a desolate stretch of the interstate when suddenly we heard a loud thudding sound and the car began to shudder. We immediately pulled over to the side of the freeway and discovered that the back tire on the passenger side had gone flat. We looked for a socket wrench to remove the lug nuts, but there was none to be found. We ended up leaving the car by the side of the highway, and walked to the safety of a grassy field to wait for a tow truck. Katherine and I sat down in the grass and gazed upwards at the pitch-black sky that held billions of shining stars. We watched, awestruck, as one shooting star after another blazed its way across the darkened screen of the night sky. It was August, and the magnificent Perseid meteors were strutting their stuff. Our inconvenience changed in that instant from a royal pain in the ass to a magical mystery tour.

The stars had always been there, waiting patiently for decades until the two of us finally came to a stop, looked up, and took notice. That August night we did stop—or did something stop us? I'd wondered for a good many years whether the things that happened to me were a coincidence, or whether they actually happened for a reason. The more I thought about the events in my life and other people's lives, the more I became convinced that things do indeed happen for a reason. Those reasons often remained hidden from view to be revealed to us only at a much later date. I came to agree with Kierkegaard's observation that "life could only be understood backwards, but must be lived forwards."

When I thought about that dark August night, it was as if some unseen, indescribable force stopped us, wanting to show us something. Now it was my cancer that had stopped us. No more zipping down the highway of life at full speed. That night I saw the golden strands of my daughter's hair for the first time.

"Bad Horsey!" my daughter-rider shouted as I balked, not wanting to go towards the imaginary barn. "Bad Horsey!" she repeated, attempting to prod me forward by sticking her bare feet spurs into my reluctant ribs.

I tried to put my all into her cowgirl saga, but my all was only about one-third of what it had been before. Plus, my mind refused to stay in the moment, preferring instead to wander off and worry about what would happen next.

I WAS SCARED when I went alone to the Cancer Center the next morning. The grim agenda that day was to run through a "simulated" radiation treatment.

I didn't have long to wait before the doors opened, this morning to reveal Rick, a clean-cut man who looked young enough to be a high school homecoming king. He explained that he was the radiation tech who would be helping me that day. There was a light, smooth jazzy feeling to Rick's demeanor, and there seemed to be no worries in his young world, no threatening storm clouds upon his horizon. He asked me how my earlier experience with the CT scan had gone and I recounted the story of Leon and the missed vein.

"Bummer!" he replied.

We ambled through the clinic, walking past the various offices of the staff. One office belonged to the clinic physicist, the person who would ultimately be in charge of designing the computer program for the conformal radiation I would receive. Conformal radiation was a relatively new development in the field, and I was lucky to be at a university that helped pioneer it.

We continued our tour into what Rick described as the treatment area. "One of the techs will come out to get you in the waiting room and bring you here," he explained. We entered the men's dressing area, a small room featuring two sets of lockers on each wall and two wooden benches. "Just strip down to your skivvies, put one of these gowns on, tie it in the back, and we'll come and get you. And that's that," he said in his carefree voice.

If only that were true!

No worries, Rick promised—there would be no treatment that day; all they would be doing is "taking some measurements" for my treatment and running "a simulation."

My blue jeans would have slipped off by themselves if I hadn't cinched them tight into the very last hole of my belt. I'd already lost a waist size or two from the chemo. I fumbled around as I tried to tie the stupid blue and white cotton gown behind my back. I never did understand why people couldn't wear the darn thing tied in the front.

I heard Rick knock on the dressing room door. He walked me down the hallway past a room with a red flashing sign above a door that said, "DANGER-RADIATION." Rick explained that the door led to a treatment room, and that the flashing sign meant that someone's treatment was in progress. We walked by the red light, continued to the left, and stopped at an open doorway.

"Here's the control room," Rick said.

The dimly lit room looked like a scaled-down version of the command bridge on the starship *Enterprise*. Two technicians sat in front of large panels with various monitors and an assortment of buttons and dials.

The two technicians introduced themselves and explained that one of them would be in charge of administering my daily treatment. They assured me that I would be carefully monitored when the radiation was administered, and pointed above their consoles to a smallish window that looked down into the treatment rooms. They couldn't let me look through the window because a patient was in there, and they needed to protect his privacy.

Rick and I then waited back in the hallway. I cringed as I heard a faint buzzing noise coming from behind the door during breaks in our conversation. After a few minutes, the red sign stopped flashing, and one of the technicians left the control room, pushed some more buttons, and unlocked the door so we could enter the treatment room. I was impressed by the thickness of the door as it swung open. I assumed that it was lead-lined to keep the radiation in the room.

A second technician came into the treatment room carrying a two-foot-square piece of pea-green plastic mesh. He dipped the square into a silver pan filled with water, removed it, and pressed it against my face until it morphed into a mask. Once the mask was formed, they cut out two small holes for my eyes and one for my mouth. The techs explained that I would need to wear the mask when I received the radiation to insure that my head would not move—not even a millimeter. No one needed to tell me what would happen if the destructive rays hit my eye or my brain.

I looked at the cast as the techs wrote my name and date of birth on a white tag and attached it to the mask. Was that all that would be left of me at the end of the day? What if things went haywire in the control room and the radiation machine was mistakenly commanded to nuke me? I visualized a smoking mask, lying empty on the treatment table.

My morose imaginings were interrupted by a tech asking me to hop up and lie down face-up. The tech instructed me to move "just a hair" this way, and that—to the left, right, up, and down. The techs were assisted in their endless measurements by another in the control booth, who I assumed was looking at the images of my sinister tumor on a computer. Once I was lined up to their satisfaction, they placed the freshly minted mask over my face, attached the sides to the treatment table with large bolts, and screwed my head down tight to the table.

I looked past the intensely focused faces and busy hands of the two young technicians and tried to check out the room. The treatment room was cavernous, and the control room window stood approximately fifteen or twenty feet above the floor. The top third or so of the walls were lined with shelving that held row after row of green mesh masks with white tags, the casts of the faces of my fellow victims. Who were they? Where did they live? Who did they love? I hoped that they had someone like Katherine in their lives.

KATHERINE

GREG GOT UP EARLY and was out of the cottage before my eyes were barely open. He wanted to check out the local gym in Dexter, and go from there to the radiation clinic for his first trial run. He was my morning guy. I fumbled with my fears as I kissed him good-bye.

Emerson and I started setting up the cottage, and I began to think about making connections to the community. We drove into Ann Arbor and discovered Hands On, a children's museum in the heart of downtown. After an introductory tour, Emerson returned to the play kitchen and immediately set to work. Her housekeeping fantasy with the plastic fish, wooden bread, and tiny dishes was insatiable.

My mind returned frequently to Greg. I imagined the ordeal he must be going through, lying alone on a table, trying to hold his handsome face perfectly still. Thankfully, there were only a handful of children in the museum that day. I found a quiet spot next to Emerson in her make-believe kitchen and closed my eyes. My love flew to Greg. The connection was powerful and undeniable. Emerson and I left her kitchen and headed home to prepare some real lunch.

GREG

I HEARD THE SOFT BEATS of the techs retreating footsteps, followed by a loud thud as the lead-lined door shut tightly behind them. The bright lights in the room dimmed, and I could see the two technicians hunched over the console in the backlit control room. "We're going to begin now," came the disembodied voice over the intercom loudspeaker. I summoned up whatever courage I could, raised my arm, and gave a thumbs-up. "All right," the voice replied, "we'll have you out of here in no time."

"No time" is an expression other people use when describing your feeling of "forever." I believe it must have begun in the medical field, probably in a dental office. I lay painstakingly still, screwed tight to the table, waiting…waiting…wondering what the hell was going to happen next.

"Just a minute," said the no-time voice. "We have to make some adjustments."

I raised my thumb again. Better now than later, I thought, remembering that the best carpenters measure twice so they only have to cut once.

"All right. We're ready. Here we go!"

All of sudden a whirring sound came from my left as the machine next to me came to life. It actually looked pretty goofy, like a gigantic telephone handset with an oversized earpiece. It began to circumnavigate my head, stopping at different locations determined by the program designed by the physicist. The top of the machine contained several disc-shaped areas that looked like the floating heads on an electric razor.

At each stop around my cranium there was a series of clicks as the heads rotated and the lenses changed their focus. I was scared out of my mind! How on earth would I be able to handle being bolted to a table and blasted every day for eight weeks? The masks on the shelves looked down on me like ancient skulls in a cave. What was I thinking when I agreed to do this? I must have been nuts!

What if I'd actually lost my mind some time ago, and all of this—the cancer, the crazy doctors, a death ray machine that looked like a piece of space junk left over from a budget science fiction movie—was some kind of nutty, psychotic hallucination? I'd seen many people on the psych units over the years that lived in different realities. Several of the patients swore they were Jesus. One patient speaking with a pathetic imitation of a British accent claimed to be John Lennon. Another person swore he was psychic and knew where Jimmy Hoffa was buried.

I never thought that I would wish to be psychotic, but that day, when my head was bolted to the table, I had a new appreciation of why people took refuge in la-la land. Still, I was sure I didn't want to be anyone else; I wanted to be me.

KATHERINE

WHEN GREG APPEARED AT THE COTTAGE DOORWAY, I dropped the book we were reading and ran to him with Emerson close behind. As the three of us embraced, it was difficult to know who was holding up whom. I felt a tremor pass between us as we lingered there, clinging to one another.

After a simple lunch, we drove across the lake to a small public park with swings, slides, and a fishing pier. Everything was still wet from the morning rain, but Emerson didn't care and neither did we. She ran back and forth between us, picking dandelion stalks stripped of their flowers or seedpods. She clasped the bouquet of green stems and exuberantly presented them to her daddy. It was his first gift of flowers. In the shadow of Greg's cancer, we saw the preciousness and fragility of life everywhere.

That evening our friend Parker drove from Grand Rapids to join us for dinner at the cottage. He and Greg had been great friends for the past twenty years and their connection was deep. I knew bits and pieces of their history, such as how Parker's mother-in-law used to bake pies for them and they'd eat the whole thing in one sitting. I knew their friendship had sustained them during the arduous years of graduate school. Greg had been an entertaining companion to Parker when he cared for his infant daughter while his wife worked.

That night Parker's six-foot frame towered over Greg, and they both cried as they embraced. I was overcome by their unguarded display of tenderness. I happily served Parker tofu curry, steamed

greens, and grape juice in place of our usual glass of wine. We talked, eager to catch up, and then finally were off to bed. Each of us was
preparing in our own way for tomorrow and the unknown it held.

The morning arrived with the welcome sunrise over the small ex-
panse of silver water. We purposely distracted ourselves; Greg and
Parker went to try out another gym in Ann Arbor, and I escorted
Emerson to the public library, then back to the Hands On Muse-
um. When the two of us headed back for Emerson's afternoon nap,
Parker shepherded Greg to his first radiation treatment.

I knew Greg and I couldn't do this alone. We needed the whole
universe. Every clear act would have to be done with love and intention, free from attachment or rejection. That was our path.

10.

THE GOOD FIGHT

GREG

THE SUN SEEMED BRIGHTER than normal the following afternoon as we wound our way through the country roads toward Ann Arbor. I squinted as rays of sunlight muscled their way through the trees and into the car. There was an unfathomable, palpable power that came from the sun, our life-giving star, and I was painfully aware of the consequences of overexposure after being sunburned too many times.

I was about to get blasted with ultra-high doses of concentrated radiation, which I knew couldn't be good for anyone. The technicians would hide in their lead-lined fortress, while I was to be bolted to a cold silver platter, wearing nothing but my skivvies and a paper-thin hospital gown that I couldn't even tie!

Parker and I entered the radiation clinic, and the cheerful receptionist greeted us. A radiation tech escorted me to the men's locker room. Two other men in gowns sat on the bench, staring at the floor. They appeared deep in thought.

It felt like I was in an elevator; a small space where strangers exhibit feelings of awkwardness. I decided to try to break the oppressive silence by acknowledging each of them with a simple, powerful greeting, one that I knew only the most obstinate or autistic could resist.

"Hey, brothers," I called out.

The strategy worked like a charm. The three of us took turns introducing ourselves and briefly describing our individual battles. They were veterans of the cancer war, and they had the battle scars to prove it. The men were thin as rails, with fiery red skin. I asked them what the radiation had been like. While my new brothers mentioned some side effects they'd experienced, they both said that it "wasn't too bad." I knew they were lying, but I also realized they were trying to protect me. I would learn the truth soon enough.

My tech arrived, escorted me into the treatment room, and instructed me to sit on the table. He grabbed a long pole with a curved hook on the end, then reaching high to one of the shelves, he snatched my green mask and lowered it to the table. Another tech joined him and introduced herself. Mary was a tall woman, whose long dark ponytail was secured by a colorful sequence of hair ties.

Mary and I talked as she and her teammate carefully positioned me on the table and bolted my head down. I made an extra effort to reach through my heavy curtain of gloom to establish a more personal relationship with the techs. I figured that if I expressed an interest in their lives, they, in turn, would have more of an interest in mine and be extra careful to push the right buttons on the control panel.

Mary told me she had two children, including a boy the same age as Emerson. She asked some questions about who I was, and when I told her about Katherine and Emerson her face expressed compassion.

You can tell a lot about a person by the way they touch you, whether it's in the form of a handshake, a hug, or even a pat on the back. Touch reveals a person's character, and can often give you a snapshot of their truer, deeper self. I can tell the moment that I shake a new patient's hand if they are skittish or fully present, weak or strong, scared stiff or courageous. No matter how hard you try, you can't control your autonomic nervous system. I could tell from the way Mary's hand rested on my shoulder that she truly cared about me.

She wished me well as she and the other technician left the room and shut the door behind them. I was alone—well, sort of. Right next to me was the radiation machine, and a light on it was blinking. I thought about the movie *Goldfinger*, and James Bond getting strapped to a steel table in a spread-eagle position. A giant machine shot a deadly red laser beam that cut a steaming hot line through the table heading straight toward his crotch.

There I was, strapped to a table, about to be blasted. The laser-like beams aimed at me were trying to kill the villain that was part of me. Too bad some special agent with a cool gadget or souped-up car couldn't save me! My hero was back at the cottage, playing with Emerson.

The heads of the technicians reappeared in the window of the control room. Mary raised her arm and waved at me, and I gave her a thumbs up in return. The room darkened, and I could feel all 640 muscles in my body tighten in anticipation.

The arm of the radiation machine began to spin slowly around my head, then came to a stop. There we were, face to face, examining each other. The lenses of the machine made a clicking noise as they rotated and tried to find the right aperture through which to shoot. As I looked up at the rotating heads, I knew I had to find a way to change my thinking and see the machine not as my enemy, but as an ally. As the treatment began, I shut my eyes tight and visualized the power of the sun coming down through the machine to heal me.

KATHERINE

I STRETCHED OUT ON THE FLOOR of the cottage while Emerson napped. All I could think of was Greg. Several hours had passed since he and Parker had left for the Cancer Center, and my thoughts repeatedly turned to him, just twenty miles away. I closed my eyes and immediately saw the cancer invading and destroying the man I loved. I was overcome, unexpectedly, with a great rage and it filled me with righteous power. My heart began to beat fast, preparing me to fight. I wanted to hurt it, smash it, and rip it out of his body!

Then I stopped and looked more carefully. The cancer was primitive and embryonic. It was the antithesis of our life—devoid of purpose, consciousness, even malice. It had no plan. We needed to respond to it with swiftness and clarity. It did not belong in our life. Greg and I were here to serve, to teach, and to fulfill our life purpose with love.

Angry again, I focused my thoughts like a samurai and destroyed the tumor with deftness and thoroughness, severing its roots. In my image, one strong taproot remained. I envisioned water rushing in and flushing out the tumor from its very base. There was a flash of brilliant light, and the water flowed clean and clear. There was true intention, soulful and heartfelt, where the tumor had once been. I knew that somehow we would prevail. We would not cower in front of cancer or its treatment. Thy will be done.

I sent the truth of my visions to Greg. Through all the challenges that would follow, he would find his true self. This was his time. I fell into a light sleep. I never told Greg about my visions; I didn't need to.

GREG

THE LENSES ARRIVED AT THEIR PROGRAMMED STOPS, and at each one there was a loud series of buzzing. The death rays were shot into my skull rapid fire, faster than an automatic machine gun. Finally, the clicking noise of the rotating lenses stopped and a man's voice came over the intercom. "How we doing?" I didn't know how he was doing, but I was a mess. The rays were not painful; the only thing I could feel was my heart pounding against my chest wall. "We're gonna finish up now," the voice continued. "We're almost done." I closed my eyes tighter than before as I sent a silent prayer to an unknown god, "Please get me out of here."

The heavy door opened and Mary came over to the side of the table, quickly loosened the bolts, and removed my green mask. She smiled as she looked down at me. She reached out and touched my hand.

"You did great," she said.

"Yes," I replied, as if doing great meant that I had lived through it.

She helped me off the table. My legs were as shaky as a toddler's trying to stand for the first time. I thanked her as she led me down the hallway to the door of the dressing room.

"See you tomorrow," she said cheerfully as she left me at the door.

I dressed quickly, and met up with Parker. We didn't talk about the treatment as he drove home to the cottage. I didn't want to think about what had just happened to me, or what was going to happen during the next eight weeks. Instead I changed my focus and our conversation to his new (used) car, a gorgeous black 700 Series BMW. Sinking into the warm, leather seat couldn't have felt any more different from lying on the cold table in the sterile radiation clinic.

The sound of cool jazz from a Detroit public radio station drifted softly from the car stereo. I pushed my thumb against my ears, alternately blocking off each ear to see if I could still hear out of both sides. The music and Parker's voice flowed smoothly down each ear canal. I breathed a sigh of relief as I realized my hearing was still okay. A much bigger test followed as I covered my left eye and could clearly make out a cell tower off in the distance with my right eye.

Good enough! I put my trembling right hand over my right eye and cautiously opened my left. The cell tower hadn't moved an inch; it was as plain as day, sitting up there on the hillside. I was so happy! I hadn't died that day and neither had my left eye!

KATHERINE

THAT DAY ALONE with Emerson gave me precious time to reflect. Was there a word for the magic that we needed for Greg? I thought about the relatively new field of research known as psycho-neuro-immunology—a complicated word describing how the mind and the emotions, the nervous system and the immune system talk to each other and are inseparably connected. What I had believed for forty years was being scientifically confirmed: The power of our emotions and our thoughts become amplified through the channels of nerves, neurotransmitters, and hormones, and influence how cells function. What goes on in our hearts and minds matters! It boils down to the fact that when we are unhappy or stressed, our body, especially our immune system, doesn't function optimally. The converse is also true—when we are experiencing love, beauty, and connection with life, our immune system is enhanced.

As a fourth-year medical student, I applied for a small grant to design a six-week independent study of holistic medicine. It meant lots of extra work doing original research and writing a thesis, but I was hungry for the opportunity. It was 1975, when it was uncharted territory. I was thrilled when I was chosen out of dozens of applicants.

I had identified three centers in the Midwest that I would visit and report on. One was a progressive cancer center located outside of Chicago. It has survived many transitions, and is known today as the Cancer Center of America. The center integrates traditional oncology care with complementary therapies. While there, I was introduced to "guided imagery." A traditionally trained radiation oncologist, Carl Simonton, had pioneered it just a few years earlier. He was convinced that a patient's state of mind could influence his or her ability to survive cancer. Guided imagery used relaxation and visualization as tools for survival. Over the ensuing years, Dr. Simonton became known throughout the world as the granddaddy in the field.

I was asked to assist in teaching these new techniques to patients. I had my own life struggles and had come up with my own images, but I didn't want to oversimplify the process. It couldn't be orchestrated like a paint-by-number kit, so I encouraged patients to find their own images, metaphors that resonated deeply with their own life stories.

Over the ensuing decades, I continued to believe in the power we all possess—an innate ability to tap into our own unique images for healing and recovery. I have presented these ideas to the hospitals where I've worked, to assist patients going through surgery as well as those in our cancer groups. The research was clear. Patients who used guided imagery techniques needed less pain medications, had fewer complications, and shorter hospital stays. Nonetheless, no doctors from surgery or anesthesiology would show up when we presented our ideas. Not to be discouraged, I would meet personally with them and lobby to get a pilot program going. After multiple attempts at our local hospital, I worked out the logistics so that patients could learn about guided imagery. Preparing for major surgery is like training for a marathon. Listening to guided imagery tapes prior to, during, and after surgery improves outcomes. Hospitals around the country have been given financial support and reimbursement from big insurance carriers, including Blue Cross and Blue Shield, for using guided imagery techniques.

Greg and I tried some imagery together when he first learned of his diagnosis, and we listened to tapes while he was going through his second round of chemotherapy. Lying beside him with the tape player between us was helpful, but I could sense it "wasn't his way," and he balked at the structured exercises. It felt contrived to him. It was like the seat belt that he wore; he resented it because it constrained him. He abhorred anything that had too many rules or steps. His Sagittarian mind preferred the straight shot of the arrow, not all the details.

Yet I still believed it would be helpful for him to connect in some important way with the cancer, or to feel its presence in his body. I knew it was a difficult thing to ask, but he agreed to try.

Greg closed his eyes, and after guiding him through a gentle relaxation exercise, I asked, "What do you see?"

He paused for several minutes before he finally said, "I see swirling lights."

I asked him to explore further, "Ask it to speak to you."

He began to cry. "It's dark now," he said through his tears.

I reached out and held him, and we didn't talk. I knew he would find his own images and their meaning in his own time. What I didn't know was when and how his image would come to him.

GREG

WE DROVE IN THE COTTAGE DRIVEWAY and both my eyes noticed that someone had given the grass a fresh cut and trim. We promised Sue that we would take care of the lawn, but I hadn't had the time or energy to find anyone to do it. It was odd that someone had cut it, but my thoughts were already on Katherine and Emerson. They ran into my arms as tears streamed out of both my eyes. Somehow, we had made it through that first horrific day, but I was sure I couldn't make it through another eight weeks.

Emerson climbed up on me, her imaginary horsey, and rode me to the vet. "Horsey sick," she explained to her vet self. She had me turn over on my back and held her careful hand on my stomach. "Tummy ache?" she asked, and I nodded my head and neighed yes. I was well aware that children work out their issues through play, but as I swallowed the imaginary pill she gave me, I realized I was also hard at work on mine.

When Emerson touched me that early evening I felt the touch of a true healer. She gave me the best medicine in the world—love. "All better!" she pronounced, and I quickly turned my face into the carpet to hide my tears. She had said the magic words that no one else could utter, the only words that would release me from my slow but sure demise.

I COULD BARELY SUMMON THE ENERGY AND COURAGE to go back to the radiation clinic the next few days with Parker. It was a major struggle just to get myself out of bed and force down my protein shake in the morning. Now it was time for him to return home, and when his BMW pulled out of the cottage driveway, I was sure I had seen him for the last time. We both tried to be strong as we said goodbye, but his sad, compassionate eyes revealed the truth we both knew. My dying was now a question of when, not if.

My dreams were becoming more disturbed and much more difficult to understand. They were a jumbled, swirling combination of violence, rays of flashing lights, and feelings of terror. I wondered if my nightmares were a side effect of the Klonopin I had been taking, or the result of all the stress I was under. I surmised that there was a vicious war going on inside my head, and I was always the victim.

The radiation treatments the next few days followed a predictable rhythm: frustrated attempts trying to tie my stupid gown, techs bolting my face to the table, and the intermittent buzzing of the machine gunning its intense rays into my face. The only noticeable difference was that the two men whom I had first met in the dressing room were gone, replaced by two new patients who were just starting their treatment. I wondered what had happened to the men in my original group. Were they too frail to continue? Did they die? It felt like we were a squadron of fighter pilots, and one by one cancer was shooting us down.

As a psychologist I believed in the "power of positive thinking," but now there was no way I could deny the grim reality that faced me. I struggled to hold back the growing tide of my despondency. I tried to maintain an upbeat, we-can-do-it game face for Katherine and Emerson, but my fear and depression were so strong that I could no longer pretend. My tiny bit of energy and optimism disappeared. My psychic dam caved in.

After Parker left, it took some doing to convince Katherine that I could still drive myself to the clinic, and before she could rescind her reluctant blessing, I climbed in our Subaru. As I began to pull out, I noticed Luke standing next to a beat up Econoline van in his rutted dirt driveway. I rolled down the window, stuck my hand out, and waved. Luke responded by walking quickly over to my car.

"How ya doin' with all that cancer stuff?" he asked, wrench in hand.

"I'm doing fine," I lied. "Just gonna' get some more radiation," I explained, like someone going to the grocery store to pick up a quart of milk. "You know, some days it's radiation, some days it's chemo."

"Holy shit!" he exclaimed. Luke summed it up perfectly.

It occurred to me that Luke was being a lot more honest with me than I was with him. I asked him if there was any chance he had seen anybody mow our lawn, as I wanted to make sure that I paid him.

"You ain't payin' nobody!" he declared, pointing his wrench at me. Suddenly his taut poker face gave way to a wide smile. "I did it!"

Twenty dollars would have gone a long way for Luke and his family. Normally I would have jumped at the opportunity to pay him, but I held back, knowing that if I offered, it would have put a damper on his pride. Instead of money, I offered my gratitude.

"Thanks, brother!" I said.

"No biggie," he replied, yet his beaming face told me a different story. It was a huge deal to me too, one that I thought about during my reluctant drive to the hospital that day. The interaction with him that morning reminded me of the creature that Dr. Frankenstein created who became a vengeful "monster" only after it was denied the love and acceptance it so desperately needed. Even though the book was science fiction, I watched that horror story come to life time and time again during the remembered childhoods of my patients. People aren't born angry; they become angry after they are hurt.

What happened to Luke? Was he ever loved? Who hurt and rejected him? How did he express his rage? Did he ever have friends who brought him into their garage and encouraged him to throw plates full of anger against a wall? Whatever he may or may not have done in his past, he sure didn't seem like a monster to me that morning. Luke and I may have come from different sides of the track, and it was true that we were fighting different battles that day, however, the deeper truth was that he was a brother, one much more like me than different from me.

KATHERINE

THAT NIGHT, GREG AND I settled into bed and slept. I dreamt that I had a tumor and was telling the news to my partners, Nancy and Sharon. I explained that I needed to leave them.

I woke up, and wondered what the dream meant. Then I remembered my recent decision to break away from my medical practice. How was it that Greg and I were simultaneously facing such cataclysmic crossroads? We were both being asked to fight for our lives, for what we really believed, and to demonstrate our commitment through our choices and actions. For a moment, I doubted myself in the dark morning hours, yet I knew there was no going back.

Despite all the uncertainty, I decided to stay connected with my patients and return to the office one day a week to attend to them and their medical needs. This meant leaving the Silver Lake cottage every Thursday and working a full day at my office on Fridays. Taking Emerson with me would also give her time to reconnect with her life back home and her Montessori friends. I hated leaving Greg, even for a short stretch each week, but it was the best arrangement I could come up with. We needed to leave a path back to our future.

Thursday came and I drove reluctantly down the dirt road, leaving Greg in the hands of Parker. Sadness swept over me, even though we would only be separated for 36 hours. It felt like eternity. Pushing away, I felt the solidity of the nest we had built at the cottage over the last few days. Greg would return home to Traverse City on Friday when his treatment was over.

Once the tires met the paved asphalt, I felt the pull of my other life. Emerson had a swim lesson, and I was scheduled to introduce a guest speaker from Duke University who was coming to town for our Lecture Series. The four-hour drive home was filled as we immersed ourselves in the books-on-tape that I'd borrowed from the Ann Arbor library. We giggled at Amelia Bedelia and her escapades. I created elaborate stories involving Emerson's dearest imaginary friend, Dorothy from *The Wizard of Oz*. Dorothy was lost in the woods, but was quickly found by treehouse fairies riding acorn caps in the river. Emerson's imagination was as deep as my love. This was my tightrope. It kept me present and stretched 200 miles across the Michigan peninsula.

Back home, I turned my attention to a huge stack of papers from the office while Emerson napped. The house was empty and I felt disconnected. I'd forgotten my cell phone and, horror of horrors, my hair dryer. But it was so much deeper than these inconveniences. I heard what people said, but I couldn't connect; my heart was elsewhere.

A vague feeling of déjà vu crowded in on me. Hadn't I done this before? I was standing in the shadow of someone threatening to leave me. I was being punished. I didn't know what I had done wrong.

I began to cry, I was sobbing as I remembered how it felt years ago. I was a junior in high school and drove my thirdhand car, a white Renault, back and forth to school. But that day I wasn't going to school; I was going to my mom's apartment where she lived with my brother. It was just a few miles from our family home where I lived alone with my father. I went to check on her because she sounded troubled over the phone.

My mother was one of the most intelligent human beings I've ever known. She had a strong passion about things that mattered to her: civil rights, women's rights, my rights. True, she was not the voice-rising, foot-stomping type, but she wasn't afraid to take the difficult road. She'd left my father and supported herself as a paralegal in a law office. She wasn't afraid or too busy to talk to my friends about things that mattered to them. She supported a friend of mine who chose to have an abortion when she got pregnant her first month at college.

The summer before, we'd taken a trip to the Smoky Mountains of North Carolina. It was just the two of us, and we read our favorite poems and stories out loud as we drove north. Yet, this was the same woman who had struggled with mental illness since I was eight years old. Her illness would come and go like an unwanted guest, and I seemed to be the first to know when it arrived.

I knocked loudly, and when no one came to the door, I entered her apartment. The room was dimly lit. I found my mother disheveled and agitated. The dishes were piled up in the sink. She told me my brother had lost his temper the night before, scattering newspapers on the kitchen floor, then throwing things from the refrigerator at the wall. He had left for the day. Her words became more and more random, and I had trouble understanding what she was trying to say. Something about Russians and how they were trying to send her messages at the grocery store.

She began to recount a conversation with her coworker at her office. The woman was describing the dinner she'd made for her daughter and her new son-in-law, but somehow Mom knew that all of the talk about food was really about sex. She was exasperated by everyone's confusion and preoccupation with things that didn't matter. She began crying and talking about how she didn't want to live anymore. She wouldn't answer me when I spoke directly to her; she just looked into the distance somewhere over my shoulder.

I decided to call her psychiatrist to arrange for an emergency appointment. Somehow we filled the hours as I tried to reason with her and to stop her from thinking about hurting herself. Nothing I said connected or registered with her delusional mind.

I was exhausted by the time we arrived at her appointment. I walked with her into the psychiatrist's office and introduced myself. I explained how she was feeling suicidal, and how we had just spent the last six hours. The doctor looked at me over his bifocals. "Young lady," he said, "have you thought about this? Now, who is the mother and who is the child?" The doctor was scolding me!

I stared back at him in disbelief. I was too stunned to be angry. "No," I answered, bewildered, "I haven't had that luxury." I couldn't believe this professional was accusing me of being the problem. My mother was ill, and I was doing all I knew to do.

I stood there, looking at him, unable to speak, and feeling that somehow I had done something wrong. But how could I possibly be the one who was guilty? Why was I being punished? I didn't want to remember, but it all came back to me.

During my first semester in college I went to visit Mom in her new apartment in Virginia for Thanksgiving. I took the train from New Hampshire where I'd been working as a teacher's aide, part of my college work-study program. When Mother picked me up at Union Station, she was so preoccupied and disoriented she could barely drive. Later that day she fought with me as she tried to leave her apartment half-naked to make a statement to the world. She was desperate to share her message.

There was no turkey that Thanksgiving. I spent my holiday having my mother admitted temporarily to the psychiatric ward at the local hospital, against her will. I spoke on the phone to her older brother, Walter, and explained the situation. He instructed me to empty out her apartment, box up her things, and have her committed to the state hospital permanently. I was horrified by his suggestion and refused. I still believed in her and her ability to heal.

Now, here I was in Traverse City, staring blankly at the kitchen counter covered with a pile of papers. I had to face the possibility of losing my best friend and husband to cancer. I felt once again that I must have done something terribly wrong and that I was being punished. For some irrational reason, I connected losing my mother with the impending death of my husband. The two events were juxtaposed like two photographs, out of order, in some scrapbook.

My adult mind couldn't sort out the breaking heart of my child. Of course, with my mother I would have preferred to be the child rather than the mother and now with my husband I wanted to be the wife and not the doctor. But my choice was not on the menu. Resistance would serve no one. Maybe feeling guilty was my way of making some sense of it all. At least, in that way, someone was responsible for the tragedy. That someone was me.

GREG

KATHERINE DECIDED WITH GREAT RELUCTANCE to leave the cottage for a quick overnight trip back home so that she could attend to the needs of her neglected patients. I tried to reassure her that I would be "fine"—something we both knew wasn't true. What went unsaid was that this was likely a dress rehearsal for our final act together, when, lying on a hospice bed, I would tell her that she must go on and live her life without me.

So this is how it will all end, I thought as I watched the taillights of Katherine's aging Subaru bounce up and down the dirt road back toward Traverse City. I slid down into the couch and fell into a bottomless well of despair. Katherine had lovingly prepared my dinner, the usual protein shake, and left it on the table, but I just couldn't bring myself to get off the couch and drink it. Now I could see why people give up and let go, waving their white flag of surrender.

I thought about my tumor, the ravenous monster that was foraging through my head at that very instant, destroying any healthy cells in its path. My thoughts returned to all the patients I tried to help on the psych units over the years, basically good folks out of hope and control. As I closed my eyes, I imagined my imminent death and visualized my memorial service. Mercifully, my pain and Katherine's suffering would soon be at an end. I tried to convince myself that dying would actually be a good thing, as it would finally release Katherine and Emerson and me from this nightmare.

I grabbed the television remote that was on the sofa. We had not watched TV since arriving at the cottage, but I needed something to distract what was left of my mind. I pushed the power button on the remote. An image of two African American boxers appeared on the oversized screen. One of the boxers was dressed in white shorts, his opponent in black. I rubbed my eyes, refusing to believe what I was seeing. Yet there it was, in living color—the "Rumble in the Jungle"—the same Ali-Foreman fight I had seen in the documentary *When We Were Kings*! There was Ali, against the ropes, his gloves raised to protect his face, as Foreman pounded his abdomen with heart-stopping fury. Ali dropped his gloves briefly, and Foreman seized the opportunity and drilled Ali's left sinus area. At the same instant that Ali was hit in his face, blood poured out of my left nostril in a bizarre and dramatic synchronicity.

As Foreman continued to pound Ali against the ropes, the African fans began their chant, "Ali, Ali, Boma ye." An epiphany came to me, and I fell to the couch, sobbing uncontrollably, struck down by the power of my realization. Not only did I know what was going to happen to Ali, I knew what was going to happen to me! It was as if I were in the white shorts and the tumor was in the black ones. I continued to weep as I was struck by the realization that the cancer would not kill me, but that I would kill the cancer! Ali and I had become fused in some weird, metaphysical double helix that defied reality.

KATHERINE

I RECALLED THE WORDS OF A SPIRITUAL TEACHER, "Your trials did not come to punish you, but to awaken you—to make you realize that you are part of Spirit and that just behind the spark of your life is the flame of infinity." I offered my mother's psychiatrist to the flames. I offered my uncle. I offered all my suffering and martyrdom. I was waking up. There was more to reality then the one in front of my face. I was not being punished. I was not guilty. I had done nothing wrong.

I lowered my head onto the stacks of paper and let myself cry. I remembered a book by Carol S. Pearson that I'd read twenty years ago, *The Hero Within*. It describes six archetypes that we, as part of the human collective, use to define ourselves: the Innocent, the Orphan, the Wanderer, the Warrior, the Altruist, and the Magician.

I have always felt a resonance with the Orphan archetype and my upbringing, or rather my lack of upbringing, as a young girl. And I have felt a definite pull to be the Martyr with my bottomless response to the hardships of others, including just about everyone I've ever loved—my mother, brother, father, and my first husband, not to mention all my patients. Pearson suggests that there comes a point in our life when the role is mastered and we move on. I remembered the day I felt completely finished with the martyrdom path and literally said to myself, "I am no longer loyal to the suffering."

But what was I now? Did I need to become a Warrior? Me? What was a warrior anyway?

I'd had my share of fighting. When I was eight, I beat up the young boy in the neighborhood for looking at me the wrong way. I fought to stay in the newly desegregated high school when all my friends dropped out to get their surrogate diplomas from a GED program. I fought for my integrity during medical training. Yet I always believed that there was a better, "higher" way of being than fighting.

But I could not deny that what I was up against now was a real fight, and I was playing for all the marbles. I was facing the biggest challenge of my career at the same time my husband was facing off with the world's deadliest cancer. Where were my boxing gloves?

How could I fight both at the same time? I was athletic, but was never involved in competitive sports. I was smart, but not the debating type. Who had prepared me to fight? As I combed my memory, I came up blank.

Maybe I was thinking of fighting in the wrong way. Maybe it didn't need to involve blood and bruises and violence. Hadn't I quit smoking after being raised by two heavy smokers and fifteen years of my own addiction? Hadn't I left a difficult marriage? Didn't it count that I left a well-paying job when I outgrew it? Weren't all of those *fights*? I even told my mother a few years ago that she couldn't visit us if she didn't take her medicine. And once, I hung up the phone when my dad accused me of being selfish because I didn't want to rescue my brother.

The word "courage" came to mind, and I remembered it was derived from the Latin *cor*, or "heart." It means doing things from your truest convictions, from your *heart*, from the *core* of who you really are. It doesn't mean you aren't afraid, but it means you do difficult things in the face of your fear. And who had been my coach through difficult times? Greg! The very person I had to fight for now. I would take the stance of the Warrior.

GREG

THE PHONE RANG. It was Katherine, calling to see how I was doing. I could barely hear her voice above the screaming African fans as they stormed the ring. Ali's booming voice came across the room in surround-sound, "I am the greatest! I am the greatest!"

"How are you?" Katherine repeated.

"I'm great!" I yelled into the phone as the blood continued to gush out of my nose. "I'm bleeding!"

"What?" Katherine asked.

"I'm great!" I repeated. I tried to explain what was happening, but it was impossible. All that came out of my mouth was a manic jumble of words.

Katherine was frightened at my sudden onset of profuse bleeding, and berated herself for leaving me. I tried unsuccessfully to convince her that I really was great and encouraged her to stay where she was. We said our goodbyes with a great reluctance. I stepped out the French doors, walked to the end of the dock, and looked upward into the sky. My epiphany began to disappear behind rapidly increasing clouds of disbelief, skepticism, and embarrassment.

I tossed and turned that night as I went over and over those bizarre few minutes on the couch. There was no way in hell I would ever tell the doctors in the Cancer Center what had just happened. I was sure they would put me on some kind of anti-psychotic medication. I imagined how the whole thing would go down:

"Let me see if I have this straight, Dr. Holmes. You believe that a TV talked to you and gave you some kind of message about your cancer? How often do you hear voices that other people can't hear?"

Maybe the tumor had destroyed part of my brain and I was going nuts after all. But in the end, I was bound and determined not to let go of what had happened to me that night. I held onto it with a viselike grip; I refused to throw my towel into the ring.

KATHERINE

AS PLANNED, I LEFT EMERSON with a babysitter and went to the local college to introduce a speaker at the Integrative Medicine Series I had organized. I was exhausted. I could think only of all I'd had to go through just to show up and perform in this parallel universe. As I tried to straddle my two worlds, I hit my head on the edge of the car door. It throbbed with pain.

Before the talk began I slipped into the lobby to call Greg from the pay phone. It was a poor connection. Greg sounded agitated, and said something about his nose bleeding. There was so much static on the line, I could barely hear him. I reached up to my forehead and noticed there was blood on my fingertips.

Greg seemed excited, and tried to reassure me that he really was "great" and that he would explain it all to me later. I was worried about the bleeding and could barely concentrate. Only twenty-five people braved the pouring rain to attend a lecture that wasn't very good. The whole night was a disappointment. People said I looked tired and I was. I dug deep to find my warrior.

11.

FLOW

GREG

ON MONDAY KATHERINE AND I WENT TOGETHER to the radiation clinic to meet with Dr. Abdul and assess how the radiation treatment was progressing. His nurse weighed me in, and Dr. Abdul made note of the obvious—I was losing weight. He asked how I was "tolerating" the radiation.

"I don't think it has affected me all that much," I replied.

His eyes and his pen remained fixed on my chart as he uttered his terse reply, "It will."

I wanted to believe that going through radiation would be different for me, that the rays would destroy the tumor and leave the rest of me alone. Katherine was doing everything she could to help my body withstand the toxic treatment. She spent countless hours researching alternative medicines, preparing various supplements, and making the protein shakes that I hated to drink.

Leaving the radiation center, we made our way over to the cancer clinic for a follow-up visit with Dr. Francisco, my chemotherapy oncologist. His physician assistant, Mary Beth, met with us and discussed the results of my recent PET scan. I burst into tears when she told us that the cancer had not metastasized or spread to any other area of my body. She responded to my outburst with a quizzical look, and I quickly explained to her that it was the first "good" news since I'd been diagnosed.

Dr. Francisco came in the room, looking his dapper self. He wasted no time performing a quick review of my chart, as well as the fresh measurements taken by Mary Beth. He was unimpressed by the PET scan results, remaining concerned about the cancer spreading into my lungs, but conceded that there was no evidence of lung cancer "yet." He explained to us that the purpose of the chemotherapy was not so much to kill the cancer, as to "soften up" the tumor for radiation.

Tears filled my eyes as I asked Dr. Francisco if I would survive. He deflected the question by retracing the ground he'd already covered. Simply not enough was known about this rare, aggressive tumor to make a clear prognosis, he said.

But I pushed on and pleaded, "Is there any hope?" I so badly needed to know before enduring more torture from the radiation.

The million-dollar question hung in the air between all of us. Dr. Francisco looked down at the floor as if searching for a trap door to escape through. He continued to be evasive, preferring to stare at his highly polished brown penny loafers rather than return my gaze.

"We're doing everything we can," he said. He wished me good luck as he escorted me from the room.

KATHERINE

WHEN WE RETURNED MONDAY TO THE CANCER CENTER in Ann Arbor, I realized we'd been wise to make the push to come home on weekends. While we were home, a restorative change came over Greg. Caravanning back to Ann Arbor, we felt replenished, and Greg believed he could do this terrible thing that lay in front of him.

I watched him stride with determination through the door into the treatment room as Emerson and I settled down to play in the waiting room with the same toys I'd noticed a week earlier. I put my heart into the moment as my two loved ones did what they had to do. Emerson discovered many of the toys had pieces missing, but that didn't stop her from pouring herself into the Sesame Street dollhouse. Who said this eyeless potato head couldn't be Big Bird's friend?

An hour or more passed. Finally Greg pushed through the doors that separated us and shuffled across the room to where we were both sprawled out on the floor. He seemed distant and I felt the "radiation cloud" had come over him. I was no psychic, but viscerally I could feel it. His spirit was exhausted, injured in some invisible way. He collapsed beside us in an empty chair and ran his hand over his almost hairless head. He leaned down to tie his shoe. Every movement seemed to take such effort. We gathered our things and stepped into the cool, early evening air.

Dr. Francisco could not have been more discouraging that day, but I buoyed myself with positive thoughts about everything I was doing—juicing food for Greg to eat, making smoothies, praying, journaling, researching supplements, and caring for all of us. I remembered my consultation with Dr. Leichtman; I heard his voice tell me over and over to "Go for broke!"

I was initially overwhelmed when the nutrients I'd researched and ordered began to arrive on our front step. Now I needed to come up with a schedule for Greg to take them. They couldn't all be swallowed at once, and many of them needed to be given on an empty stomach. How many times a day did Greg have an empty stomach?

The plan I came up with was elaborate and ambitious, but with the help of my friend Kate, a masterful organizer, I brought it in to focus. The hour-by-hour regimen was first handwritten on a piece of poster board, then typed up, copied, and laminated. I placed the

CLEANSING COCKTAIL

Can be made with a juicer or blender. A juicer extracts juice and removes most of the pulp and fiber. For a thicker consistency, consider using an industrial blender, which blends the entire food into a juice/smoothie.

- 4 carrots
- 1 apple, cut into wedges
- 2 celery ribs
- ½ cup parsley
- 2 beets (with tops)

instructions in the kitchen, and bathroom, and in the baskets we used to transport them to the cottage.

I tried to relax and make light of my efforts. Was this some weird scavenger hunt? Had I gone over the edge with a full-blown obsessive personality disorder? Yet I truly believed in this "madness." These nutrients would be our good friends, powerful with their unique medicines to help him.

I wasn't kidding myself; I knew it was also a way to feel like I had some control. I prayed that it was helping. People said he looked great—and he did to me on most days. Clear, radiant, loving—even more than usual. Yet I told myself that even if there was no response, it was not a failure. I recalled Alice Bailey's teaching, much of it too esoteric for me to understand, but one passage stood out in my memory. She instructed that in healing work we must do everything we can with love and wisdom and then step back with no attachment to the outcome. Not having an attachment to Greg's outcome seemed impossible, yet I knew it was, ultimately, what I would have to do.

My job was to keep each day as fresh and intentional as I could. Most days I even discarded hope because it was a distraction from the present moment. It was like throwing pennies into a deep well, wishing for some hypothesized future or some remote past. By hoping for something different, I would miss the reality surrounding us.I didn't want to prepare for a future that might not contain Greg. I told myself that I could handle it, but could I really? Would I want to? I understood the teachings of the beloved Vietnamese monk, Thich Nhat Han better—the best way to take care of tomorrow, is to take care of the present moment. How precious was the sound of Greg's footstep in the hall, his voice on the phone, his strong embrace, his Subaru in the driveway? I reminded myself to touch these deeply, to savor his perfect presence.

Later that evening, we discovered a small Middle Eastern restaurant downtown. We sat outside under a blossomed redbud tree complete with heart-shaped leaves and small, delicate flowers. I watched Greg out of the corner of my eye, and was relieved to see he was able to eat small bites of hummus and tabouli. Seriousness came over him, and for a few minutes he sat there deep in thought. Then he turned to me as Emerson chattered, and confided that he needed someone to talk with, to help him emotionally and spiritually. He wiped his mouth with the napkin from his lap, then said sadly, "I'll call John." He was referring to a therapist he'd known and trusted from has days as a graduate student. I nodded my head and gave him my blessing.

SCHEDULE FOR GREG'S SUPPLEMENTS

Upon Awakening

- MCP powder (see pages 52–53)
- Maitake or PSP mushroom extract (see pages 205–207)

Before Breakfast

- Proteolytic enzymes (page 223) with:
  - Curcumin (page 181) 500-1000 mg of phytosome curcumin complex
  - Quercetin 200-400 mg (page 152)
  - Silymarin (milk thistle) 150-250 mg (page 153)
  - Green tea extract ECGC 250 mg (page 154)
  - Grape seed extract 100 mg (218)

With Breakfast

- Whey shake (see page 38)
- Probiotics
- Omega 3 oil from fish or krill (total per day 700-1400 EPA with 400-800 DHA)
- High dose multivitamin with antioxidants (Vitamin C 1000 mg, Vitamin E with all tocopherols 400 IU, and additional tocotrienols 50–100 mg)
- Vitamin D (get blood level checked and supplement to achieve level of 50-80 mg/dl)
- Coenzyme Q10 100-200mg

Before Lunch

- Proteolytic enzymes with quercetin, curcumin, grapeseed extract, silymarin, green tea extract

Lunch with organic veggies, lean protein, as appetite will allow

- Additional Vitamin C 500-1000 mg and omega 3 oil
- High dose multivitamin with antioxidants (Vitamin C 1000 mg, Vitamin E with all tocopherols 400 IU, and additional tocotrienols 50–100 mg)
- Coenzyme Q10 100-200mg

Before Dinner

- Fresh juice or green drink
- Proteolytic enzymes with quercetin, curcumin, silymarin, green tea extract, grape seed extract

Dinner with organic veggies, complex carb, lean protein

- High dose multivitamin with antioxidants (Vitamin C 1000 mg, itamin E with all tocopherols 400 IU, and additional tocotrienols 50–100 mg)
- Coenzyme Q10 100-200mg

Bedtime

- MCP and Maitake or PSP mushroom extract
- Melatonin 20 mg* **

* www..nebi.nim.nih.gov/pubmed/22753734

** For how and why melatonin is an effective cancer treatment see www.naturalnews.com/033511_melatonin_cancer.html

QUERCETIN

Quercetin is the most common flavonoid in the human diet. Flavonoids are plant-based compounds with powerful antioxidant properties found in fruits and vegetables. Quercetin is especially high in apples, onions and tea. Growing research is accumulating about quercetin and how it influences the cycle of cell growth in cancer. The unique thing about quercetin is that it exerts this growth limiting effect on cancer cells and not on normal cells.

Its value to cancer patients, other than being a great incentive to eat fruits and vegetables, is that it has been shown to induce cell death in cancer cells (apoptosis) and to decrease expression of the mutant p53 gene. This healthy gene is important as it suppresses tumors.

Great scientific articles describing the effects of quercetin include:

- Review Article: "Quercetin and Cancer Chemoprevention"; Lara Gibellini et al

- *Evidence-Based Complementary and Alternative Medicine,* Volume 2011, Article ID 591356, 15 pages

- http://www.cancer.org/treatment/treatmentsandsideeffects/complementaryandalternativemedicine/dietandnutrition/quercetin

SILYMARIN (AKA MILK THISTLE)

Milk thistle is a plant that originated in the Mediterranean but now is found worldwide. It is a tall plant with purple thistle flowers. The most well studied component of this herb is the flavonoid silymarin. Research suggests that silymarin protects the liver from toxins, including aceteminophen (Tylenol) which damages the liver at high doses and the poisonous mushroom(Amanita phalloides). There are potential benefits for repairing the liver from alcohol and Hepatitis C. As an anti-cancer therapy, research suggests that it has the following potential properties:

- Anti-inflammatory
- Growth inhibition
- Cell cycle regulation
- Inhibition of angiogenesis (blood vessel growth)
- Apoptosis (cell death) induction
- Inhibition of invasion and metastasis

Great reference on milk thistle and cancer is http://www.ncbi.nlm.nih.gov/pmc/articles/PMC2612997/

GREEN TEA EXTRACT

Green tea is famous for containing many polyphenols (compounds from plants that contain many ring like structures or phenols). EGCG is the most studied polyphenol in green tea. It has been shown to inhibit every step in the creation and growth of cancer. These include:

- DETOXIFICATION. Stimulating phase II enzymes in the liver that make carcinogens less toxic and less able to create cancer.

- DNA REPAIR. Green tea will stimulate repair of damaged DNA. If too much cell damage has occurred, apoptosis (or cell death) will be encouraged by EGCG.

- INHIBITS GROWTH SIGNALS. If a tumor is already present, green tea makes it harder for the cancer to spread by slowing down the growth.

- REDUCES ANGIOGENESIS. Green tea slows down the process of blood vessel growth (angiogenesis) and blood flow to the tumor.

How much do we need to drink to get these effects? For cancer prevention, at least five cups per day. For those with known cancer, ten cups per day. It is estimated that each cup of tea contains 50mg. Green tea is also available in capsule form. New formulations have combined the green tea extract with phytosomes to enhance absorption.

Greg received 250 mg three times per day. Our goal was to protect his salivary glands, skin and immune system during radiation treatment and to enhance the cancer cells response to radiation therapy.

GREG

I FELT WEAK AND KNEW I WAS DROWNING FAST. In desperation, I dialed the number of the therapist I had seen years ago while completing my doctoral training. John had proven to be a real lifesaver once before in my life, when I was trying to survive the treacherous waters of an extremely dysfunctional and abusive doctoral program. Although the program had been highly rated, I soon discovered there was danger lurking below the surface. I'd heard rumors when I started my training that my major professor had a serious mental illness, and it wasn't long before I experienced his sickness on a firsthand basis. His mood swings proved to be as wild as they were unpredictable; any innocuous comment made at the wrong time would set this brilliant man off on a wild tirade. His office was in constant disarray with papers and books strewn everywhere; it was literally impossible to see a square foot of carpet as the floor was littered wall to wall with journals, interdepartmental memos, the remains of yesterday's lunch, and unidentifiable junk. He would often forget our scheduled meetings, or he'd suggest we hold meetings in his trash-filled van while he raced across town to pick up dry cleaning he'd forgotten the week before. The scariest part of his erratic behavior was that he was the professor I had to depend on. He was supposed to be a mentor to me, the one to show me how to become a good psychologist. Yikes!

I would have left him for another faculty advisor, but in our small department it was verboten to switch horses in the middle of the stream, even if your horse was grievously sick. Whatever problems you had with your major professor were seen as *your* issues that obviously stemmed from *your* childhood. The grave consequences became crystal clear when I expressed a reluctance to pursue some crazy idea my major professor proposed for my dissertation. He became enraged at the thought that I just might have some ideas of my own! He threatened to "blackball" me at the university if I refused to do his bidding.

John, an adjunct professor in the counseling center, was the antithesis of my nutty professor. His caring, consistent presence and level-headed nature were a much-needed antidote for the school's toxic environment. Although John never spoke of it directly, faith was at the core of his beliefs. He seemed to embody all that was good about religion or spirituality; he walked the walk rather than just talking the talk. I hoped he would help me deal with my despair and guide me along the gentle descent toward my final destination. I wasn't looking for a cure; I knew that was wishful thinking. I just hoped that John could help me with some guidance at the end of my life.

He answered my call with the same jovial voice I'd grown to treasure. He seemed genuinely happy to hear from me, and was distressed to learn I had cancer. Unfortunately, he had retired several years ago and couldn't meet with me as a client. We talked about my belief that I needed to find some spiritual guidance, and he suggested a number of books I could read that might be of some help. He told me it had been an honor for him to know me and work with me, someone so bright and talented. Although I appreciated his gracious comments, his use of the past tense had a haunting effect. I knew it would be the last time I talked to John, and, even worse, I knew it was the first of many goodbyes to come.

KATHERINE

THAT NIGHT GREG AWOKE AT 3 A.M. and couldn't get back to sleep. He felt the nausea growing and his appetite slipping away as anxiety consumed him. I didn't know what to do, and then I remembered acupuncture. He had responded positively to my efforts in the past. Why not offer his body calming, nurturing energy?

I fumbled in the bedroom darkness and gathered my acupuncture supplies from my study. Greg stretched out in our bed and I uncovered his arms and legs. With only the nightlight to guide my hands, I took his pulse and inserted the needles. They were almost painless, and he barely winced as I placed them. I chose points for reducing the fire in his body, nurturing his blood, and quieting his heart. His breathing deepened and his pulse became stronger and slower. It seemed to calm him and comfort us both, as we tapped into this ancient healing. We both took a quarter of an Ambien pill. Sleep was so precious now—a time to just be and not worry or think.

In the morning light we discovered the trees surrounding the lake were dressed in new clothes—a fresh vibrant green. A man fished from his small boat as it drifted on the still lake surface. Greg sat beside me, writing. He stopped mid-sentence and looked at the clock. It was a few minutes after eight and his treatment was at 8:50 a.m.— it had been just fourteen hours since his last one.

This time, he said he'd go alone. He wanted Emerson to have a chance to catch up on her sleep. I offered him a small mountain of supplements and he made a face at the sight of them, but mumbled, "Thank you." Then I handed him the whey protein shake and attempted to entice him with the fact that the concoction had fresh strawberries in it. He winced, but once again said, "Thank you," and hugged me with his arms full. I watched him drive down the dirt road. I lingered, listening until the car's engine was a distant purr.

The week of treatment passed quickly, and before we knew it, it was Thursday and I was driving north again for the other life. Emerson went to school, I worked, and Greg returned alone on Friday night. He arrived home before us and stood in the doorway with his arms open as we hustled to join him. We had made it through the second week of treatment!

GREG

I SPENT A LOT OF TIME THAT SUMMER in our maroon, 1998 Subaru Outback, which had been my loyal companion for several years. I nicknamed her "Flow" in honor of her ancestor, another Outback I'd purchased years ago from a fisherman who lived on the other side of the state. I found the first Outback in the classified section of an obscure shopping guide. It was already several years old, but what intrigued me was the unusually low mileage for its age. When I called to ask about the car's condition, the owner seemed insulted by my question, and threw down this gauntlet: "If you can find a scratch on the car, I will give it to you!" There was something intriguing to me about this man, and I needed to check it out.

I was so excited about the car that I left immediately, arriving early evening at the modest, yet well-cared-for farmette. Jim was a tall, older man who held his eyes in a constant squint, even though the sun had already set. It was clear from the start that Jim was a no-nonsense, all-business kind of a guy, with little time to waste. "Let me show you where she is," he said, as he spun on his beat-up Red Wing boots and marched toward the barn. Jim slid open the large wooden door and we were greeted by the pleasant smell of hay. In the middle of the barn sat the car—buried under several layers of old newspapers. "Let's get to work," Jim demanded, and we began to remove the newspapers like two archeologists, digging through layers of civilization, hunting for buried treasure.

As we scraped away the mound of papers, Jim explained that the buried Subaru had been his wife's car that she'd purchased several years ago when she had "the cancer." She needed a reliable car that could make if from their farm to the hospital for her chemotherapy. She passed away just a few months after her treatment began. Jim paused for a moment in memory. "I just couldn't sell her car after she went. She loved it so." I asked Jim what his wife's name was. He replied, "It was Florence, but she favored Flo. So that was all there was to it. That's what I call her." I noticed he used the present tense when he talked about his departed wife. A part of him still refused to believe she was gone.

The car gradually revealed herself, and she was indeed a beauty. The phrase "mint" condition couldn't do her justice—she was pristine. There may have been a small scratch or two on her, but I didn't have the heart to look that hard or to confront Jim. I knew that he was letting go of much more than a car. We both stood quietly, gazing down at the car, like a family looks at a loved one before the casket is closed.

When I registered the Subaru in my name, I decided to purchase my first vanity plate. I knew immediately that I would have the prisoners stamp FLOW on the plate, both in memory of her previous owner and my growing fascination with the psychological phenomena known as "flow," as described by the psychologist Mihaly Csikszentmihalyi. He believes that when a person is experiencing flow, they are completely immersed in an activity during which they often feel great joy, at times rapture. This was in contrast to feelings of depression and anxiety, signs that a person was not in the flow.

I had witnessed so many of my patients over the years resist going with the natural flow of their lives, only to suffer disturbing consequences. These were the people who went against their intuition and ignored the red flags planted in the sands of their psyches. The young people, for example, who pursued a career path for their parents instead of themselves; the people who wrote off their sour stomach on their wedding day as "just a normal case of the jitters"; the people who forced themselves to stay in jobs they hated because they were afraid of change.

I watched again and again as people struggled in vain to deny their own truth. What they really wanted to do, who they really were attracted to, who they really were. At times I would point out the window of my office to the Boardman River. I would remark that, yes, it was possible indeed, with great effort, to swim up the river. But before they jumped in, I would caution them; the unseen current was much stronger than they could imagine, and sooner or later the river would win and wear them out. Then I would suggest they imagine jumping in the river, going with the current—the flow—and how it might feel to float without effort.

Flow proved herself to be a great car for many years, but the salty winter roads of northern Michigan were too much for her in the end. A cancerous rust began as a tiny bubble under the paint of the left side of the rear wheel well, then multiplied rapidly and spread through the rest of her body. Her heart, the engine, remained strong until the very end, just as I imagined Flo's did, and just as I imagined Jim's would. It was my heart that was breaking now.

12.

PANDORA'S BOX

KATHERINE

MY BODY ACHED and the left side of my back was becoming increasingly painful and tight. Emerson still insisted that I carry her on my left hip, and the hours of driving back and forth to Ann Arbor were having their way with my body. Saturday morning I rose early to go into town for a massage and to grab some private time to reflect on the events of the week.

As I stretched out on the table and started to relax, I recognized a familiar pattern in my body and psyche. I felt that the earnest little girl of my past was still trying to fix others in a way that only covered up my pain. With the help of the massage, I let it all go and was surprised to discover a true strength coursing from my torso into my legs. Beneath the effort and strain, there was a power that connected all of me. I felt deep gratitude for this time to focus and heal.

"Thanks David. That was just what the doctor ordered!" I said with a grin.

"Want to call Bernie?" David asked.

My lifelong dream included joining with other healers to practice together under the same roof, and over the past year David and I had talked about working collaboratively. We had even looked at real estate together. Now David and I looked out the window and across the lot at the house next door. The publishers of *The Healing Garden* magazine currently occupied it.

I remembered the first time I'd gone inside the building to introduce myself to the staff. I'd felt the building was calling me. Really! I walked through the rooms and sensed that I had finally found the future home for my office. Sure, it was creaky, and the bathroom was the size of a postage stamp, but there was something greater that spoke to me.

After I left that day, I called Greg. "I think I found my office!"

"Great!" he said, "Is it for sale?"

"No," I replied.

"Is it for rent?"

This time I hesitated before I answered. "No, I don't think so."

"Well then, how could it be your office?" Greg was puzzled, but not critical.

"I don't know, I just feel it's the place."

The phone was silent for a few seconds, but I was sure I could hear him smiling.

"Fine," was his only response.

That was some months ago. Since that time I'd spoken with the magazine people about the availability of the building, and they'd explained that they rented the house on a month-to-month basis from a man named Bernie who wintered in Florida. David and I had tried to call him on the phone once before. When no one answered, I left a message.

Now David asked me again, " Do you want to call Bernie?"

"Sure!" I felt invigorated and confident after the massage. I dialed the number on the sticky note saved in my wallet.

This time a brusque voice answered. It was a man's voice. I introduced myself and asked if Bernie was there.

"Yes, this is Bernie Soucha," he grumbled.

I quickly explained my interest in the little grey asbestos-sided house on Front Street, and asked if it might be for sale.

Bernie paused, and then said elusively, "Yeah, I could consider it, but I don't know. I'll be back in Traverse City in a few weeks. Call me then."

I was so excited I wanted to scream, "You bet I will!" But instead I kept my cool, quietly wrote down his local phone number, and said goodbye. I had trouble believing what was happening. How could I simultaneously experience joy and elation while feeling such despair and depression?

I got home in time for breakfast and discovered Greg and Emerson were playing some silly game about "poopy diapers." Emerson had been toilet trained for over a year, but she loved to discuss the messes her stuffed animals found themselves in. Both of them were relieved to see me. Greg seemed preoccupied even when I told him about my adventure in town. I understood—how could it be otherwise? I wanted so desperately to make things different for him, but sometimes, like now, I just needed to let it be.

Later that same day, all three of us headed into town so Greg could walk at the gym and Emerson and I could visit the co-op. Shopping there usually included an encounter with a kindred spirit who I hadn't seen in ages. Sure enough, as soon as Emerson was settled into the small seat in the grocery cart, I noticed a good friend Anne across the aisle. As soon as our eyes met she came over, eager to catch up. She was unusually animated, and excitedly told me she'd heard about my pending move through the grapevine. I was taken aback, reluctant to talk about it in public. Not yet. Not here.

In that moment I thought about Greg with his tremendous vulnerability and uncertain future. The unfairness of it all came crashing down on me. As I began to tell her about Greg's cancer, I was totally caught off guard by how angry I felt. I was sick and tired of acting like everything was okay. It wasn't! It was horrible! The cancer was inflicting sadness into our lives, into Greg's body, and our hearts and minds.

It made me so mad! To both of our surprise, I burst out, "Fucking purposeless cancer! Why? We need Greg! Emerson needs her father! I need his companionship into my nineties!" Poor Anne! She stood there listening to me rant with tears brimming in her eyes. I simmered down, and she reached over and put her arms around Emerson and me. She promised to make time for a visit with us next weekend. She wanted to help in any way she could. She offered to play her harp for Greg and maybe do some imagery work. I thanked her for listening, and I told her I would speak to Greg about it.

We drove home in silence. As soon as the groceries were unpacked and put away, I reached for little Emerson and picked her up. We headed downstairs and put *Mary Poppins* into the VCR. I loved the formality and magic of Mary Poppins' world. Cuddled together under the comforters, we slipped into the sidewalk with Mary and Bert, rode on the carousel, and chased the fox until bedtime.

A LOW LEVEL, EVER-PRESENT, PANIC SET IN. There was a fire in our house, unseen termites, or some stealth robbery happening in our midst. Whatever it was, it was stealing Greg's life away, bit-by-bit. The invisible enemy filtered into my days and crept in my dreams. I continuously asked myself what I could do that I wasn't already doing. I loved him, believed in him, and did everything I could think of to balance the devastating effects of his treatment, yet I kept feeling we needed to do more. Meditation, yoga, more acupuncture—seeing some other healer, perhaps? I watched as the sun began to set on his precious life.

I decided to telephone Libby Slocum, a well-known acupuncturist who lived in Kalamazoo. A respected person in our community had heard about Greg's situation and gave me her name. Libby and I talked about her work and Greg's discouraging diagnosis and treatment. She suggested specific acupuncture points that would boost Greg's immune system.

Libby described her use of low-level laser diodes that emitted invisible synchronized light directly into the body. She explained how the laser penetrated deeply into tissue and helped cellular pathways produce energy, lessen inflammation, and help the body repair itself. She had seen it work in the most difficult situations and believed it would help with Greg's treatment and his recovery. I was intrigued. I decided to keep an open mind and call the physicians who trained practitioners in its usage to get more information.

When I broached the subject of getting another consultation with Greg, he was adamant that he did not want to see anyone else about his cancer. I explained to him that I was afraid I was missing something that we could be doing to help him.

Greg looked at me with fire in his eyes. "I don't believe in what everyone else has to offer, I believe in you!" he said.

How could I argue with that? I decided to treat him more aggressively with acupuncture, nutrition, and most importantly, with love. Greg believed in me, and I needed to believe in myself.

We headed back to Ann Arbor and braced ourselves for what awaited us. In the coming week, Greg would receive his third round of chemotherapy back to back, over two days. There would be added appointments, the miserable IVs, and the ensuing nausea and fatigue. Our conversations detoured around these looming obstacles and we did all we could to stay focused on the moment. Who wanted to rush ahead?

GREG

ON MONDAY, WE TRAVELED DOWNSTATE for a return visit with Dr. Francisco. I thought about my life as the little green mileage markers flew by my window. Mercifully, I had few, if any, regrets. It was true that I had made many mistakes. People always say that they would have done things differently if they only knew then what they know now, but I call that cheating. Of course you would have played a different card in the game of life if you knew what everybody else was going to play!

I long ago accepted the fact that I was far from perfect. Many of my patients have struggled with issues of not being perfect: not having the perfect house, spouse, children, job. I would gently remind them (and in so doing remind myself) of the old adage, "Perfection is the enemy of the good." As we turned onto the exit toward the University Hospital, I conceded that I hadn't been the perfect husband, father, therapist, etc., but I found respite in my belief that I had been a *good* one, and that was *good enough*.

I first met with Dr. Francisco's physician assistant, Mary Beth, who genuinely seemed to care about how I was "handling" the chemotherapy. It was difficult to tell her the truth—to be honest about things not tasting right, admitting that I had lost weight, being up-front about how I felt so fatigued. Saying these things out loud made it more real, more painful.

I asked Mary Beth flat out if "there was any hope for me." She said she thought there was, but she really preferred to have Dr. Francisco answer those questions. She took the usual measurements of my blood pressure, pulse, and weight, and then excused herself from the room.

KATHERINE

GREG STOOD ON THE SCALE and Mary Beth watched the needle flicker until it came to rest at 148 pounds. The scale said that he had lost some 30 pounds, but no one seemed to notice he was wearing hiking shoes and blue jeans. Mary Beth examined Greg and reviewed his recent lab tests. We nodded our heads as she offered common sense advice about a diet emphasizing small, frequent meals with soft texture. She reminded Greg to rest and sleep whenever tired.

It was her kindness that I savored, more than her vanilla words. I knew she had seen many challenging cases and had the perspective that only experience can teach you. Maybe she could give us some direction, some hope, something to grasp on to. Would he survive? Was he doing as well or better than anyone she had seen today? Had she ever known anyone with this type of cancer? She confided that this was not her expertise, but reassured us backhandedly that Greg seemed to be "doing fine." We explained some parts of our eclectic approach. She agreed with the protein shakes and the additional magnesium Greg was taking. She seemed surprised that I knew that the chemotherapy agent cisplatin would deplete his body of this essential mineral.

Greg and I shared as much as we felt she could comprehend. I knew she wanted to be helpful and I appreciated her compassionate eyes as we described our list of supplements, testing the water of her tolerance. We only revealed a fraction of our program. I had been there before, listening to desperate people willing to do desperate things. Why was it easier to speak more openly with a nurse practitioner than it was to the physician? She seemed to have more time and less judgment. I strived to be this way with my patients; to share the power and take extra time. I wanted to go even one step further. I wanted to give specific, viable alternatives and allow them to choose.

I decided to spare her the extent of our "madness." She didn't object to any of it, yet she didn't condone it either.

GREG

DR. FRANCISCO TALKED BRIEFLY ABOUT MY TREATMENT PLAN for the week, which consisted of a double-barreled onslaught of chemo and radiation. He asked us if there were any questions, and I only had one. It was the same question I'd asked him on two previous occasions, the question that he never seemed eager to answer. "Is there any hope for me?"

Dr. Francisco twisted his tidily dressed body, uncomfortable with being put on the hot seat once again.

"Is there any hope?" I repeated quickly before he had a chance to juke me with some, "We just have to wait and see" mumbo-jumbo. I fired the question to him a third time. "I need to know—is there any hope for me!"

Dr. Francisco's face flushed beet red with an annoyance that he could no longer control. He was definitely a man who felt much better when he was in the driver's seat.

"All right!" he finally declared, as if he were confessing to committing a crime. "I guess there is always hope."

Now I was angry. What an asshole! Why was giving a simple word of encouragement so difficult for him? I felt like screaming, *Just tell me the truth! If you think it's hopeless, then why the hell are you injecting me with poison?*

But even though I wanted to yell at him that day, I held my fire for two reasons: one, I knew that it wouldn't do any good; and two, like an abused spouse, I was too dependent upon the person who was hurting me.

We didn't talk with Dr. Francisco about the disturbing truth that all three of us knew too well—that the chemotherapy was highly toxic, a poison that would race through my bloodstream, continuing to destroy my healthy cells and tissues along with the cancerous ones.

MAGNESIUM

An extremely important mineral in the human body and essential to over 300 biochemical reactions, it is estimated that eight out of ten adults do not reach the recommended daily intake for magnesium. This contributes to it being one of the most common nutritional deficiency in the U.S.

The reason for most deficiency states is a magnesium-poor diet and the side effect of medications, which was true in Greg's case. Rich dietary sources of magnesium are nuts/seeds, whole grains, dark leafy greens and chocolate. Most people need to supplement to boost their levels of magnesium to get the RDA of 300-500 mg per day. The best forms of magnesium are magnesium citrate or magnesium glycinate as they are better absorbed and have less GI side effects. Too much magnesium is known to cause loose or frequent stools.

Things that deplete the body's stores are stress, coffee or caffeine, and medications, especially diuretics. Conditions that can be benefited by magnesium include high blood pressure, heart disease, insomnia, asthma, attention deficit, osteoporosis, kidney stones, and migraine headaches.

Symptoms of being deficient include irregular heart rate, muscle cramps, constipation, irritability, fatigue, and insomnia.

Katherine and I had many times watched patients struggle and die from the side effects of chemo. Since anticipating that I would receive the treatment, Katherine had been pumping me full of vitamin and mineral supplements, girding my body for the upcoming battle. We were both painfully aware that most doctors scorned her approach. Their objection was that there was no evidence that nutritional supplements had any positive effect. Oncologists believe that supplements "interfere" with the chemo and make it less effective. Yet none of these objections could stop her. She was tenacious and wasn't about to give up now. We knew full well before we got to the Cancer Center that no one would believe in her approach, but I stuck my toe in the water anyway. I asked Dr. Francisco what he thought about my taking supplements; he responded that he "guessed" they couldn't hurt. "But," he cautioned, "you'll have some very expensive urine."

So we never told Dr. Francisco, or anyone else at the Center, exactly what we were up to. Katherine and I knew that we would be criticized at best, and humiliated at worst. It would do no good to get into a pissing match with them, or, as Dr. Francisco would put it, a "very expensive" pissing match.

KATHERINE

IN RETROSPECT, DR. FRANCISCO'S COMMENT about Greg's urine, although rude, wasn't all that shocking. I learned all about entrenched attitudes when I moved to Traverse City and took a part-time position as director of integrative medicine at the local hospital. When I'd come to town and interviewed with the CEO of the hospital, I shared with him my vision for a new approach to medicine that integrated complementary and traditional practices. He said reflectively, "You are an answer to our prayers." I couldn't believe my ears—my rebellious thoughts about medicine with a soul were actually welcome here! He commented that my picking up and coming to town without a job "took guts." Who was this man?

I loved working for John Rockwood. We developed mission statements and working committees. Our scope was wide and included the hospital environment as well as care for the people who worked there. We developed a speaker series that provided lectures to the community, and people responded by coming out in droves to the events.

I surveyed the hospital physicians and asked them what they were interested in learning. In response, I developed monthly teaching sessions for them, during which I focused on a specific nutrient or herb. These presentations were always prepared with an exhaustive literature search.

On one hand, the physicians seemed curious as more and more patients were turning to alternative medicine. Surveys indicated that more than 30 percent of patients sought out alternative care. Often, though, they were afraid to tell their doctors lest they be punished or ridiculed. I knew all about that!

On the other hand, the doctors felt threatened. More and more patients were asking difficult questions for which they had no answers.

I presented my information to the doctors in an objective, neutral tone and told them, "You don't have to endorse or refute it, just try to understand it." I believed that the doctors would at least be open minded enough to listen to different points of view from some of the pioneers of alternative medicine. I was dead wrong. I quickly learned that I was not an answer to anyone's prayer; instead I was a burr under their saddle.

I began to sense their cynicism, their condescending dismissal and even down-right antagonism. What did the environment have to do with medicine? What did art and music have to do with a patient's struggle with death and illness? Forget the talk about healing relationships! Why would anyone in his or her right mind use a plant or a light if there was a drug? Big pharmacy was their gold standard, not the lowly thousands-years-old practice of plant-based medicine. They gave scant respect to state-of-the-art breakthroughs on micro-nutrition. A gastroenterologist sneered at the very mention of probiotics. A cardiologist criticized the use of coenzyme Q10 or the importance of the omega-3 essential oil.

I arranged for nationally recognized researchers and physicians to speak to the community. These guest lecturers included Dr. Candice Pert, author of *The Molecules of Emotion*; Dr. Rob Ivker, author of *Sinus Survival*; and Dr. Leo Galland, who wrote *The Four Pillars of Healing*. But when I scheduled Dr. Perlmutter, a nutritionally-minded neurologist, the chief of neurology at our hospital refused to let him speak to the other doctors. His objections were vague. He criticized the fact that Perlmutter was conducting controversial research, giving IV glutathione to patients with Parkinson's disease, even though the University of Miami funded his research. He also objected to the fact that Perlmutter had developed a line of nutritional supplements for his patients. His biggest objection was that Perlmutter did not practice evidence-based medicine. Dr. Perlmutter countered with the fact that his work and theories were based on research articles from peer-reviewed literature. Ultimately, he was prohibited from presenting his controversial ideas at the hospital, despite the fact that he lectured at some of America's most prestigious institutions.

Although the speaker series proved popular with the greater community, the dissenting doctors got their way and the funding was slashed. The Integrative Medicine Program was not a "revenue generating center," and, therefore, it was gutted in the next budget. The program became a shell of its former self, regulated to a tiny office suite in an auxiliary building.

The message was clear; the hospital and doctors were not as interested in new ideas as they were in a balanced budget. It was another painful reminder to me that I was an outlier in the medical community.

13.

Saint Peregrine

KATHERINE

ON TUESDAY MORNING Cynthia and David came to Silver Lake to visit and help take Greg to his treatment. I'd known them for over twenty years, having first met them in a study group. This was a second marriage for both, and fifteen years later, they were still in love. Cynthia was radiant in her flowing tunics and strawberry red hair. She would playfully scold David when he made socially incorrect comments, and he would respond by dropping his head in his debonair way. Twenty-five years her senior, he was still handsome and vital with a head of thick, silver hair.

David informed us that he'd placed a photograph of Greg and me on the lap of a Buddha statue on his altar at home. David was a deeply spiritual man and embraced all religions. He was a practicing Catholic, but had also introduced us to Thich Nhat Hahn, and Sonya Rimpoche's book *The Tibetan Book of Living and Dying*. We sat beside David in synagogues, various churches, and at the table of the disciples of Hara Krishna. Each spiritual practice was complete and satisfying to him.

Greg relaxed in their unwavering presence and let himself laugh and cry. They added sincerity and depth to any conversation we shared. Chemotherapy was almost bearable with them by his side.

GREG

CYNTHIA CAME INTO MY LIFE when she was a graduate student at Michigan State. I was immediately impressed by her combination of intelligence, intuition, and compassion. There was absolutely no doubt in my mind that she had "the right stuff" to become an outstanding psychologist.

It was easy for Katherine and me to fall instantly into Cynthia and David's warm embraces, and we became fast friends. There was a large overlap of interest and values between us. Not only did Cynthia and I share the same profession, we ended up being wall-mates in an office building in East Lansing.

The major difference between the four of us was obvious to even the most casual of bystanders. Cynthia and David stood tall, at 6′3″ and 6′1″, whereas Katherine and I were vertically challenged at 5′2″ and 5′7″. David was quick to remind us of this fact. One night when we went to their house for dinner, he opened the front door and announced to Cynthia in his sonorous voice, "Cynthia! The munchkins are here!"

David was larger than life, a colorful character not at all hesitant to blurt out what he thought about short people or anything else that happened to come across his expansive mind. He was often brash, and if you focused solely on his crustacean-like exterior you could easily reach the erroneous conclusion that he was a grumpy individual who simply didn't care. However, Katherine and I were quick to discover the purpose of his crusty exterior. Like a crab, he needed a tough shell to protect his exceptionally soft interior. The truth is, he was one of the most caring people I ever met.

David was no stranger to illness: he had survived a heart attack and had undergone surgery for stage 4 bladder cancer the year before. His cancer and the subsequent treatment stole a great deal from him, and in the process it slowly but surely took him away from us. He was noticeably tired, in constant pain, and his garrulous speech lost considerable steam. I worried about David, and was afraid that he would not live much longer. My friend Marilyn was the first to go, and now it felt as if David and I were getting ready to follow.

Cynthia and David pulled into the driveway of the cottage in their "new" used car, a taupe colored 1999 Park Avenue. They had struggled for years, trying to stuff their tall frames into smaller, stiffer cars before they finally let themselves get a big car that offered space and comfort.

As we drove to the hospital Cynthia gave me frequent reminders to drink the supplement-packed protein shake that Katherine prepared. I knew full well that the shakes were my lifeline, yet I could only take one small sip every few minutes. There were raw sores in my mouth and throat from the chemo, and it was painful to swallow anything.

Before they left to go home that day, David presented me with a medallion of St. Peregrine. A friend had given David the medallion shortly after hearing about his diagnosis. David had placed his hopes and prayers on the medal, pinning it to the pillow on his hospital bed during the surgery to remove his tumor. I choked back tears when David gave the medal to me attached to a simple silver chain. It was as if he and I were teammates in a relay, and he was passing the baton to me to complete the race. It was classic David. Even though he was suffering, he continued to think about others to the very end.

I rubbed the medallion between my thumb and forefinger as I watched the big Park Avenue lumber down the dirt access road and recede from view. Some Catholics believe that St. Peregrine is the patron saint of cancer. After thirty years of dedicating his life to helping the poor and sick in Italy, Peregrine developed a cancerous wound on his leg. The night before he was scheduled to have his leg amputated, he fell into a trance during which he saw Jesus come down off his cross and touch his leg. The next morning, when

Peregrine awoke, he discovered that a miracle occurred; his leg was healed, and the cancer was gone. I prayed for a miracle for David, and I prayed one would happen to me as well. I placed the silver strand around my neck, fastened the clasp, and vowed never to remove it—no matter what happened.

KATHERINE

GREG, CYNTHIA, AND DAVID LEFT for the Cancer Center, leaving me alone with Emerson in the cottage. My buried fears returned in the shadows of the afternoon. At times Greg's illness and my fears intertwined and rose up before me, more powerful than he and I combined. I trembled, fighting the impulse to run from them.

My desire to discuss Greg's case with someone else returned. I needed to talk with a healer who had expertise in treating people with cancer in a holistic, comprehensive way. There had to be someone!

I remembered Dr. Sandweiss from Ann Arbor, a man I knew thought out of the box. We'd met several times at conferences over the years, and I reached out to him for his help. He was very concerned about Greg and encouraged us to see a woman physician in Detroit who specialized in integrative cancer care. He agreed to call her for me and would also fax over the information I'd sent him— CT scans, biopsy report, and information about the supplements and acupuncture program I'd started. He promised he would be in touch soon.

I jumped when the phone rang a week later. It was Dr. Sandweiss. He was apologetic, explaining that the specialist had reviewed Greg's case, and believed the tumor was too far advanced and unfamiliar for her to get involved. I remembered my own heart-stopping, gut-wrenching reaction to Greg's scans. I knew they must have equally frightened her. I was no stranger to doctor talk. Her polite refusal was really a way to not get her hands dirty with a hopeless situation.

Over the years, I have inherited many such cases from my traditionally trained colleagues; patients with vague symptoms and unsatisfying resolutions. These were the people like Humpty Dumpty, that no one could ever "fix." They slowed down their doctor's schedule and demanded creative thinking that took too much time. How ironic that I was now getting the cast-off from the holistic doctor? The unwanted patient was my husband!

I wrestled with whether or not to tell Greg about the incident and decided to mention it in an unconvincingly casual way. He didn't blink. He just held me and reaffirmed how much he believed in my power to help him. I cried in his arms. How was it that even now he could comfort me?

Greg's unwavering faith in me stoked my resolve to fight. I remembered my images of an unseen fire destroying our house, and the metaphor resonated with the research I'd recently found on the cellular mechanisms that propagate the growth of mutated cells. I'd read with fascination about a master switch in the body, known as nuclear factor kappa beta (NFkB), that resides inside cells, waiting for a signal to activate. It is the cells' smoke detector. Once activated, it moves into the nucleus of the cell and signals hundreds of reactions to amplify its message through DNA transcription. At least four hundred reactions can be triggered by the activation of NFkB, some of which bring forth cytokine and mediator molecules that increase inflammation. One of the biggest consequences of NFkB activation is the loss of apoptosis, the scientific name for cell death. In other words, activation of NFkB in a cell makes the cell immortal! It may be a smoke detector, but it doesn't call in the fire fighters, rather it fans the flames, creating more heat and inflammation. This was a huge breakthrough in my understanding of how to help Greg fight his cancer.

So just what triggers this powerful activation of NFkB? Free radicals, infections, and ultraviolet light, including radiation and chemotherapy! I realized that the unleashing of this nuclear regulator influences many illnesses—not just cancer, but autoimmune conditions, inflammatory bowel disease, coronary artery disease, and arthritis. The metaphor of a fire in our house was dead on! The very treatments used to treat cancer amplify cellular inflammation and add extra life to cancer cells! My fears of fire were more than justified, and my mind raced to discover an antidote. I knew that I had to find ways to slow down activation of NFkB.

It seemed obvious to me to use antioxidants and omega-3 fatty acids, but the real key was curcurmin, commonly known as the spice turmeric and used in Indian cooking to create the golden curry flavor and color. I was thrilled to discover that it is a major inhibitor of NFkB! My pulse quickened as I read about its potential to make chemotherapy more effective. I marveled that I had already been giving curcurmin to Greg several times each day since April, along with proteolytic enzymes; always on an empty stomach for better absorption. A mixture of gratitude and humility flooded over me.

THE FOLLOWING DAY our friend Russ traveled from Grand Rapids to take Greg to his second day of chemotherapy in Ann Arbor. Greg was reluctant to go to the Cancer Center alone, and I couldn't see how I would manage it with Emerson in tow. Russ had been through his own dark nights of the soul, and he knew how important it was to simply stand with us now. He was a therapist by trade and a fisherman by heart. He drove Greg to the University Hospital and sat with him in his quiet magnanimous way as the chemotherapy dripped into his friend's frightened veins.

The morning passed as Emerson and I entertained ourselves for the first time in front of the television. We snuggled together on the couch and watched *Sesame Street*, the antidote to all young fami-

CURCUMIN

Curcumin is the orange pigment in tumeric (the main ingredient in curry*). Benefits include it being a potent antioxidant, anti-inflammation, quenching free radicals, activation of Nrf2 and assisting the liver in detoxification.

The difficulty with curcumin is its poor bioavailability—what you swallow isn't absorbed into your blood stream and can't enter your tissues. Fortunately, a formulation has been created to remedy this. When curcumin is attached to phosphatdylcholine, an essential component of cells, absorption is increased 20-fold over standard curcumin extracts. It has been patented and is known as Meriva.

* It is one of the most biologically active and studied constituents in the botanical world. Curcumin affects almost every known target or molecule involved in cancer.

References:

- http://ar.iiarjournals.org/content/30/6/2125.abstract

- http://www.cancer.med.umich.edu/news/curcumin-improves-treatment-2011.shtml

lies' challenging lives. I indulged in a momentary fantasy that we were just a "normal" mother and daughter having a free morning at home. She was happy, and even more so when we walked to the park. She whisked off her sandals and zipped down the slide on her belly, barefoot and laughing. She was immune to the reality of our situation, and it was a contagious resilience. Soon I, too, believed in the goodness of our life. We ran to meet Greg and Russ back at the house in time for lunch. I made a simple meal of soup and tuna melts, which, surprisingly, Greg was able to nibble at. He told me the night before how he could not bear the sight, much less the taste, of cooked vegetables, and today their absence was silently celebrated.

Russ sat with Greg on the small dock in front of the cottage and they caught a dozen or so bluegills. It was a dance that thrilled us with its whirr of casting, the perfect silence, and then the surprise of each catch. He expertly released each small fish back into the warming water of late May. His companionship was good medicine for Greg and our family. Maybe life was a lot like *Sesame Street* after all. Greg rested on the day bed in the late afternoon light while I gave him another acupuncture treatment. As I placed the needles, I thought of a good friend's recent advice for my recurring states of worry. She'd simply said, "In place of worry, love. Just love him. It is so much more helpful."

14.

FIRE IN OUR HOUSE

KATHERINE

THURSDAY CAME WITH A FLURRY of activity. We had just finished packing the car when our oldest and dearest friend, Jim, arrived. He would spend the day with Greg while Emerson and I headed back to Traverse City. Tomorrow, Bill would arrive and drive Greg home for the weekend.

I looked at Greg with his energetic friend beside him, and I knew he was fading. His eyes rested on me longingly as I drove off in the fully loaded Subaru. Damn it! Why did our lives have to be so complicated? It took us five hours to get home because of the notorious Michigan spring road construction.

Friday was a Herculean day of work for me. It took all the self-discipline I could muster to get through a full schedule of patients. On top of that, there was the catching up on all the unattended paperwork from the previous week.

After I saw my last patient, I sat down with my partners, Sharon and Nancy, for a business meeting. I asked them to make some concessions for the time I would be away while Greg was in treatment. In quiet, unwavering voices they told me what they were willing to offer. I steeled my heart to what they would say; I had so little to offer back.

They told me I would still have to pay 100 percent of my share of the overhead until August. After that time, I could decrease the amount to 75 percent and become an independent contractor. I looked at the calendar. It was May 28. In my business mind I knew it was fair, but to my already traumatized heart, it was a crushing blow. It was a harsh reminder that I needed to keep moving forward with my own future plans. I wasn't happy with the gestalt of the place, but at this rate, I would soon be penniless.

I thought about mundane things that day. I needed to arrange for my own health insurance, as I was on my way to independence. Once a small technicality, health insurance now had all the importance of a life raft in a storm. It was literally, at this moment, something we could not live without. Insurance never seemed like a great investment, and now I felt remorse that we didn't have life or disability insurance for Greg.

On Saturday I awoke way too early. Like most of the other mornings, I couldn't return to sleep, so I poured through the book, *Herbs and Cancer* written by the brilliant herbalist Donald Yance. The growing soreness in Greg's throat was on my mind, and I read with interest about the soothing properties of slippery elm tea. In the dimness of the morning, I took notes and made lists by the single light on my desk. I located the supplements online and ordered them.

I had arranged to meet Bernie, the owner of the Front Street house, and to walk through the property with architect and friend, Jim Elkins. As we prepared to leave the house, Emerson protested and cried out, insisting to be held. She was tired and simply wanted to stay home. But Greg was eager to join me on the small adventure, grateful to have something else to think about other than his litany of misery. Despite the cumbersomeness of our motley party, we pushed through the million and one barriers in getting to the Front Street house.

It was time to break ground, even if only in our minds. We were drawn to the house and an undeniable ripple of excitement passed through us as we walked through the potential new space.

As we drove home, I reached over and touched Emerson's flushed face, only to discover she was clearly hot with a fever. Suddenly all her protesting made sense. I carried her into the house, tucked her into bed, and tried to understand my worry. Yes, I was worried about her, but even more so about the potential exposure to Greg. Could his immune system handle a simple viral illness? Despite all of this, I kept moving forward. There was a fire in our house.

GREG

KATHERINE HAD SO MUCH ON HER PLATE during that period in my illness, what with parenting Emerson and continuing to work. Cancer struck us when she was at the very crossroads of her career. I'd watched her struggle for years to fit into the tightly controlled world of traditional medicine; it was a bad marriage from the beginning. Katherine's razor sharp mind, combined with her loving kindness, served her patients very well indeed, but the fundamentalist doctors who ran the show had little use for her interest in alternative medicine.

I felt horrible that the cancer had become the focus of our lives instead of the clinic that Katherine always dreamed of. With or without me, I wanted her to go for it, to finally be able to live her dream. I prayed that I would live long enough to see the day that she would put her love and energy into making her dream come true. I decided to talk bluntly with Katherine about the fact that she would need a place to practice after I was gone. I laid it all out on the table: aren't people who are afraid to live dead already? I really don't know if Katherine needed my blessing or not, but we agreed that she would go on regardless of my illness. Even though I was sicker than a dog, I vowed to do what I could until the day I died.

LIKE WIND AND WAVES ON A LAKESHORE, the combination of chemo and radiation eroded my body and my resolve. The pepper in my salt and pepper hair disappeared down the shower drain along with my denial and bravado. The sores in my mouth and throat were so painful it was difficult to swallow. My weight continued a steady, scary descent: 148…138…129…125. But I didn't need to weigh myself. I knew from my fatigue that I had lost muscle, and it took more and more effort to get off the sofa. I was frightened to look in the mirror; it scared me to watch myself disappear.

The doctors issued their ultimatum. When my weight reached 120, they would have to insert a feeding tube. My memories traveled to the psychiatric unit where I'd worked some twenty years earlier. I thought about the teenage anorexic girls who were threatened with feeding tubes if they lost weight. Invariably, they would dress for their weigh-in by wearing as many layers of clothing as possible. I borrowed a page from their playbook during that sultry summer in southeastern Michigan, and began wearing jeans, hiking boots, and heavy shirts each morning that I weighed in.

15.

SOUL MATES

GREG

WE RETURNED TO NORTHERN MICHIGAN for Memorial Day weekend. I had reached the halfway point in my radiation and chemo treatments, and I had serious doubts about the second four weeks.

The pain in my mouth was unbearable. Chemotherapy had destroyed the healthy cells in my mouth and throat, and opportunistic infections were beginning to take hold. The lining of my mouth changed from a healthy pink to a flaming red. My nerve endings were on fire, and it became difficult to even open my mouth.

Eating solid food was impossible, and the shakes were my sole source of nutrition. I cringed every time I heard the Kitchen Aid blender grinding away in the kitchen. The shakes had always been figuratively hard to swallow—I couldn't stand their chalky, unsweetened taste. Now they were literally hard to swallow, and the only way I could get them down was sip by tiny sip.

I didn't have any energy, but I pushed ahead anyway and continued to exercise in a literally feeble attempt to hold on to what little strength I had left. Like most cancer patients, I was told to "rest" between treatments, but that advice felt counterintuitive. I wanted to do everything and anything to stay as strong as I could. Sitting around and doing nothing made no sense—it felt like giving up! After all, a fighter can't win a fight by resting on his ass in the corner! I believed that if I sat around and succumbed to fear that I would be dead sooner rather than later.

Katherine worried when I went to the gym to amble along the treadmill, yet I knew she would worry more if I spent all day on the couch. I followed my intuition and forced myself to keep my body moving, even though I felt like a dead man walking.

I was in desperate need of a sign that I was making progress, even a tiny bit of headway, some indication that the torture was worth it. The July 1 finish line for the end of my treatment seemed light years away.

The epiphany I experienced at Sue's cottage—that I would ultimately defeat the cancer like Ali defeated Forman—faded away in my rear view mirror. At times I would touch the St. Peregrine medal that hung around my neck and think about David and his own struggle with cancer.

Of course I wanted to believe that there would be a miracle, that God or some other unknown force would end up saving me in the end. But the heartbreaking reality was undeniable. The cancer and the treatments had reduced me to a pulp and were moving in for the kill.

Once upon a time my childhood friend Bobby was the proud owner of a Magic 8-Ball. The two of us would often interrogate the 8-Ball with all sorts of questions about our respective futures. We would turn the ball over and over, gazing at its window, waiting for the white plastic die to float to the surface and reveal our fates. When we didn't like the answer, we just flipped it over for a second, even a third opinion—whatever it took to come up with the answer we were looking for.

There was only one answer that I wanted to hear from the doctors now—that there were signs of progress and some hope I was going to survive.

Bobby and I knew the ball couldn't really predict our futures, but I had a strong feeling that the doctors at the Cancer Center could see mine. Their silence spoke louder than words. They were giving me the chemo and radiation in a last ditch effort to delay the inevitable. I decided to stop asking them if there was any hope.

I read and reread the cards and letters that Katherine and I received. They were filled with expressions of love and concern, as well as offers to cook meals, babysit, and to keep us in their prayers. One card informed us that votive lights had been lit at the National Shrine of Our Lady and would burn for 60 days. I didn't have the faintest idea where the Shrine was, or who had arranged the offering, but at that point I gladly accepted any and all the prayers and good wishes I could get—wherever the heck they came from.

One special letter came from Brenin, Katherine's son, who was working in Nepal. He wanted me to know how much he thought about me, and how he felt I had been a great stepfather and friend. I was touched to read this, as step-parenting for me had been what it is for most of us—an important but often thankless task. I understood how painful it was for most children to go through a divorce, and then have some stranger waltz into their lives. I loved Brenin and couldn't have asked for a better stepson.

Messages came from people of various backgrounds and religious beliefs, all carrying an ardent belief in my recovery. Each person was confident I was going to make it. Our friends were not oncologists, yet they gave me the exact combination of medicines that I needed—hope, love, and their faith in me.

My memory, on autopilot, flew back once more to the night of the Ali-Foreman fight. I felt a weird tingling sensation in my hands. I realized that the cards and letters came from the people in my village, imploring me to kill the cancer. I imagined all of them lining the streets, shouting, "Greg, bombe ye!"

Katherine, meanwhile, redoubled her efforts to find the right combination of nutritional supplements that would stave off the destruction of the chemo and radiation. She continued to pour her heart, soul and her blender into my care. I was able, with some difficulty, to make an uneasy peace with the thin acupuncture needles she used. She was scared, yet I could feel the tremendous courage that enabled her to soldier on. There was no doubt about it; I had the best doctor in the whole wide world in my corner.

I FIRST MET KATHERINE when I returned to Michigan from Maine. The news that a Lansing hospital was looking for a psychologist to work in their family practice residency program seemed auspicious, as I had just left an identical position. During my interview with the program director, I was offered the job on the spot. I thanked him for his time and the opportunity, but told him a full-time position wouldn't work as I wanted to develop my private practice. As we shook hands to end the meeting, he made what would prove to be a life-altering and, ultimately, life-saving suggestion. He recommended I visit the other hospital in Lansing and talk to a physician there named Katherine Roth.

Katherine's office was tucked inside a dark, decaying one-story building that in a previous lifetime housed a used car dealership. I wasn't surprised that the hospital placed the family practice program in there. In a healthcare system hungry for the money generated by high-tech procedures, the lower-earning family doctor was on the bottom of the pecking order and expected to be grateful when they received a few table scraps. Specialists and sub-specialists treat family practitioners like illegitimate children. Those patients who failed to pass their wallet biopsies by the more prestigious providers were usually referred to clinics like Katherine's. Many of these rejected patients also had complicated bio-psychosocial issues and lacked the money and motivation to fix them.

Katherine greeted me in the clinic waiting room with a surprisingly strong handshake for someone so petite. Her green eyes peered out from behind wire-rimmed glasses, scanning me as I described my meeting with the director of the other program. I was caught off guard by how different she seemed from most other physicians I knew. She did not have the arrogant, holier-than-thou attitude, and there was no hint of condescension in her voice. I would soon learn that she held a deep sense of caring, even love, for her patients, regardless of their positions in life, and that she had a passionate commitment to do almost anything for them. I had spent several years with many doctors in various medical settings, and I definitely felt that I was in the presence of someone different.

The conversation during our initial meeting was enhanced by the fact that she was fluent in the language of psychology. Her own fascination with the field began when she was an undergraduate. We discussed my interest in a part-time faculty position and quickly reached an agreement that I would assist her in teaching behavioral sciences to the residents. After approval from the residency director, we were off and running.

As the weeks passed, Katherine and I consulted with each other on a regular basis to discuss the residents' progress, as well as the patients in her practice who had psychological complications. My initial impression of Katherine—her kindness, compassion, and her broad, integrated view of medicine and healing—was confirmed. Watching her interact with peers, I was impressed with her honesty and courage as she confronted colleagues whose behaviors she found unacceptable.

I would discover even more about this remarkable woman, like how she'd grown up with the burden and care of a schizophrenic mother; how her mother divorced her rigid dictator of a father and fled the family when Katherine was a young girl; and how her siblings suffered from serious chronic problems of their own. My admiration grew as I listened to her tales of survival. Here was someone, against all odds, who refused to give up. Katherine had found a way to be a light in the darkness.

During one of our meetings. I noticed a handsome black-and-white family photograph of Katherine, her husband, and their 3-year-old son. As I looked at the portrait, a startling revelation came to me that Katherine was the kind of woman I was looking for: intelligent, big-hearted, and courageous. She was my friend and colleague, and I assumed she was happily married. That day it became clear to me that I had finally found the prototype of the woman that I was searching for.

In past relationships I was attracted to troubled, withholding women who, in retrospect, had a lot in common with my mother. Initially these women seemed like perfect fixer-uppers to me, the knight in psychoanalytic armor. All I had to do was to be a good guy, love them, and their personalities would be transformed and become as innocent as Snow White's. How grateful they would be! How wrong I proved to be! What a nut ball, grandiose idea! I came to the painful realization that I was the one who had the problem: I picked the wrong women for all the wrong reasons.

I also realized that my adult life did not have to be a replay of my childhood, and at last I was more than ready to try something else. Something that might actually work.

It had been great working with Katherine, and I believed that she enjoyed working with me as well. However, other forces were pulling us in different directions. Her husband would soon graduate from his residency program, and he and Katherine were not excited about staying in the dreary, industrial area of Lansing. They began their search for a new life with an initial focus on northern California.

Katherine and her husband left for a two-week recruiting trip. After they returned, I was eager to hear how it went. I imagined she had received several great offers, given the kind of person she was.

As we met in her office, I noticed a drastic change in her demeanor; gone was her effervescent, energetic, can-do sense of well-being. She was preoccupied, worried, perhaps even slightly depressed. I asked how her trip had gone and if they had decided where they were moving.

"Tom and I... are not... moving," she replied in an uncharacteristically timid fashion. "I realized...that...ah...we...are...meant to be together."

I was surprised, as I had absolutely no idea there had been another person in her life. Katherine just didn't seem like the kind of person who would ever have an affair.

Then it hit me. There was no "affair." Maybe it was something in the way she looked at me with those green eyes—like a deep sonar signal, *ping, ping*—searching for a similar response. The "we" meant me! Suddenly her small office became even smaller. I felt lightheaded, and started having the panicky feeling I got when I drank too much coffee. Katherine caught me completely off guard by her emotional ambush. My familiar world suddenly disappeared!

She went on to flesh out the details of her confession, much like a suspect in a murder mystery who finally coughs up the particulars of why and how they did it. I listened as she went through a lengthy list: years of a difficult marriage, feeling rejected by his long stretches of silence, futile attempts at marriage counseling, her feeling that part of her would die if she stayed in the marriage, her strong intuition that we were meant to be together.

I was terrified. Of course, I too had come to the realization that she was the kind of person I was looking for...But to actually *be* with her? Someone who was married? Somebody with a young boy? I knew that I would have to have some kind of relationship with her "ex." What fun would that be? It was difficult for me to even imagine those scenarios.

I didn't know what to do next. I was caught between the imagined promise of love and the reality of my fear. Fortunately, I was able to buy some time by telling her that I would not pursue a relationship with her while she was still married. She didn't bat an eye; of course she understood, and she went on to assure me that her divorce was imminent.

During the next few weeks I spent many a sleepless night obsessing about what a complicated mess I was getting myself into. And then this dream came to me:

I'm walking through an airport, frustrated because I can't find the right check-in counter for my departing flight. After several unsuccessful attempts I finally find the right counter and take my place at the back of a long queue. The people in front of me have large suitcases and hefty boxes to check in. Suddenly, I see Katherine at the front of the queue, looking back at me, smiling. She's checking in a small package, more like the size you would take to the post office.

I didn't need the help of a psychoanalyst to understand that dream. Yes, Katherine would certainly bring some "baggage" into our relationship—doesn't everyone? I was aware of several bags of my own, and I suspected there might be a few more stowed away in the underbelly of my unconscious. But what struck me most about the dream was the diminutive size of Katherine's package compared to all the others in line. It was much smaller than my own.

Katherine did get her divorce, as promised, and shortly thereafter I got one of my own. I said good riddance to my conflicted past and chose to be with someone who truly loved me.

THE SECOND FOUR WEEKS OF MY TREATMENT began with a follow-up appointment with Dr. Abdul. Katherine and I told him about my increasing pain and deep fatigue. He actually was happy to hear that I was experiencing intense side effects from the radiation. "Good," he exclaimed, displaying a rare burst of enthusiasm, "That means it's working."

However, Dr. Abdul was particularly concerned about my weight. He reminded me of his earlier ultimatum: *keep your weight above 120 or you will get a feeding tube.* He inquired about my diet and was visibly disturbed when I reported that I had no appetite whatsoever. He asked if I had tried Ensure, the high caloric drink that the clinic nurses routinely offered me. I told him I didn't want to drink it because it was loaded with sugar. Katherine and I were aware that some researchers believe that sugar actually feeds cancer, as cancer cells have far more receptor sites for sugar than normal cells.

"Well," Dr. Abdul replied. "I've never heard of starvation curing cancer!" The phrase "end of discussion" doesn't do our session justice. Clearly, he was not the discussing type. We were there for one purpose only, to receive his opinion, and that was that.

Later I came to a fuller realization of what might have occurred during our meeting. His sardonic comment to me about starvation was thick with a sarcasm, and I believed that he took my refusal to drink Ensure as a flat-out rejection of him and his recommendations. He was pissed off because someone like me had challenged someone like him.

Thank God looks really can't kill, because I'm telling you I would have already been dead several times over. The first one to open fire at me with their optical guns was my mother, followed shortly thereafter by the Catechism nun, my girlfriend Mary Ann's parents, their priest, my major professor, and now my radiation oncologist. Every one of them had been furious with me when I failed to walk their line. To say that I was used to it just wouldn't be true; it still riled me up plenty whenever it happened, but over the years I'd learned to not take it personally.

What most upset me during that time was that no one expressed an interest in what Katherine had discovered during her research.

There she was, a physician with boundless curiosity, who had dedicated much of her life to learning what she could do to help others, and yet she was ignored again and again.

KATHERINE

LATE IN THE AFTERNOON, our friend Mike drove from East Lansing to sit with Emerson while Greg and I went to see Dr. Abdul. I confess I've never fully appreciated how important a doctor's appointment can be. I had been that "doctor" for several decades, yet had never quite understood how people prepared themselves for their visit; how they counted the days, collected their questions, and faced their fears. Now Greg and I were the patients with important questions of our own written down on a scrap of paper, tucked in the book under my arm.

Dr. Abdul's number one concern was Greg's continuing weight loss. He had lost five more pounds, and that was not counting the extra weight of Greg's now familiar jeans and hiking boots.

As usual, Dr. Abdul drove the agenda of our visit as he tapped his pen on the desk. He insisted that Greg gain weight. It was a strange mixture of a scolding, pep talk, and a physiology lecture. He explained in his accented English how nothing would taste right. How everything would hurt and be unappealing because the radiation damaged the nerve endings on his tongue. He was careful not to say they had been destroyed. Greg's taste would come back—in six months, maybe. Suddenly I understood how difficult eating had become for him, and why many cancer centers just put in a feeding tube at the beginning of treatment to spare people from this agony. I needed to stop asking Greg how everything tasted. Dr. Abdul reminded us once again that Greg might have difficulty making saliva for the rest of his life.

These seemed such small things to Dr. Abdul, yet they mattered intensely to Greg. I stuffed the list of questions deep into my pocket. How small-minded could we be as we weighed any of this against his life? I needed to get real!

The doctor examined Greg's mouth and throat and passed the scope into Greg's sinuses. In addition to the radiation damage, he saw evidence of a yeast infection and prescribed a medication, Ny-statin, that Greg was to swish in his mouth four times a day.

We were both sobered by his words and findings. A bitter mixture of sadness and anger percolated in me, partly because of the information, but mostly from the doctor's lack of compassion. There was no human connection. No acknowledgement of all that we were doing and how hard this was for us. We weren't asking for anything other than a lifting of the veil that separated us, a simple nod of the head.

As the visit came to a close, sugar came up in the discussion. Greg said that he'd read how sugar stimulates cancer cells. He explained to the doctor that he didn't want to eat the recommended bowls of ice cream because of the high sugar content.

Oncologists had been giving those recommendations to cancer patients for as long as I could remember. Nonetheless, it's common knowledge that sugar stimulates the release of insulin. Dr. Abdul had to know that insulin, in turn, stimulates cells to take in sugar, and that it increases their growth and metabolic activity. That was basic biochemistry. But did he know cancer cells had ten times the receptors sites for insulin, and that the insulin signaling was much stronger than it is in normal cells? This was exactly how PET scans work. Radioactive glucose (sugar) is injected into the patient, and cancer cells quickly take up the glucose. The radioactive tag on the glucose causes the cancer to light up and reveal where it is hiding in the body.

Did Dr. Abdul know that the average American consumes 75 pounds of sugar each year? And that all that sugar stimulates insulin release, causing obesity, diabetes, and insulin resistance! The normal response to insulin is for channels in the cell membrane to open and allow the sugar entrance. But, as the sugar load in a person rises, the cell literally stops responding to insulin. The body then responds by making more insulin, in an attempt to force the sugar inside the cell. This combination of increasing sugar and insulin levels stimulate tumor growth. Unfortunately, the more insulin, the better for the cancer.

Newer research has shown that insulin encourages precancerous cells to develop into malignant cells. This increase in insulin signaling is a necessary step in the initiation of many common cancers, particularly breast and colon. Patients with lower levels of sugar and insulin in their blood stream have better cancer outcomes.

Was this information something that I read about in some new-age health food throwaway newsletter? Quite the contrary. It was actually the results of cutting edge research from the Albert Einstein and Dana Farber Cancer Institute in New York.[1]

DR. ABDUL WAS DISMISSIVE to Greg, as expected, and I didn't say anything that day. I knew what the outcome would have been. Still, we had received the verdict from on-high, and immediately began to strategize how to give more calories to Greg without the toxicity of sugar. I thought of coconut milk and the "good oils" that come from nut butters and avocados. Greg agreed to try to eat four to six small meals a day. I knew Greg was particularly relieved that there had been no mention of the feeding tube.

---

1 *International Journal of Cancer,* July 2009; Elevated Insulin Linked to Breast Cancer; Author George Kabat, PhD, Albert Einstein College of Medicine

Journal of National Cancer Institute, November 2012: Insulin and Colon Cancer; Author Jeffrey Meyerhardt, MD, Harvard-affiliated Dana Farber Cancer Institute

A DREAM LINGERED from the night and I felt the power of the images reach into the grayness of the early morning. I couldn't go back to sleep, even though I knew I needed to rest. My half conscious mind returned to the dream:

I was carrying Emerson through the house, and discovered ink splattered on the walls, the floors, the bottom of my slippers. I had, unknowingly, tracked it everywhere. I needed to wipe it up quickly before it dried. Confused about where it had come from, I followed the inky footsteps to the edge of the room where there was a swimming pool. I saw in horror a body floating facedown in the water. After just a moment I recognized that it was our next-door neighbor, Roy. I was terrified. Should I pull him out? Call the police?

Suddenly I was wide-awake and sitting bolt upright. What was the dream trying to tell me? I had a sickening feeling that the ink was Greg's cancer! It was spreading everywhere, and there was nothing I could do to stop it!

GREG'S LIST OF SYMPTOMS WAS GROWING. The rawness in his throat made it difficult for him to swallow even the tiniest sips. His face was full of pain, and he constantly braced his hand with outstretched fingers against his left cheek in an effort to stop the throbbing. The skin under his left eye and across his face was fiery red and chapped. Our anxiety grew as we worried about what was ahead. We knew one thing for certain; there would be more pain. Greg was trying, for some unknown reason, to hold off on the narcotics. I felt frustrated, because many of the things I believed would help him he either didn't like or couldn't swallow.

Despite my fussing and his protests, I knew that the deeper problem was not what I was trying to give him; the real issue was facing the inevitable. Each additional treatment added more pain to the already grim situation.

So this was what they meant when they talked about quality of life. Before his diagnosis and treatment, Greg was "fine," other than his stuffy nose. Now his life was full of suffering. Actually, it was overflowing with it.

Of course, I understood that life was bittersweet, full of joy and suffering. When we first started I had not been able to envision the other side, the end of the treatment path. Now I knew it was all impermanent. Like how the light of day follows the night, I knew we would get to the other side of this terror we were living. Greg's treatment would not go on forever. July would come, but the next four weeks would be the dark nights of the soul.

My love was deep; it was endless. I continued to draw from my deep soul connection with Greg, and we walked the path with courage and heart. I prayed that I could move through the fears and beyond…transcendent.

Meanwhile, I faced the "circus reality" of our lives. Greg asked me to take charge of the calendar. As wonderful and priceless as the visits with friends were, they became more and more tiring for both of us. Greg had extended himself in his interactions with the fullness of conversation and laughter over the last six weeks, but pain was driving out the sweetness. He had become irritable and impatient. He needed to be silent and conserve his energy. I was also feeling more sensitive to every bump in the road. We agreed to one or two visitors each week, and requested that they only come on Wednesdays and Thursdays.

We were stripping down to the essentials. I contemplated whether it was really necessary for me to work two days each week. Every time I left it meant someone needed to transport Greg back and forth to his treatments in Ann Arbor, then bring him home. Yet I felt I needed to keep one part of my life alive and separate from his illness. With Greg, Emerson, and the long ledger of demands each day, my health and equanimity had never felt so critical. Whenever

I could, I stole moments for my pen, for my breath, and for my prayers.

I OFTEN THOUGHT ABOUT MY SON Brenin on the other side of the world. He had chosen to defer his entrance into college, opting to travel and live outside the classroom for a year. He was accepted into the Student Partnership Program, which brought young people together from different countries to work in under-developed parts of the world. Brenin was assigned to Nepal, where he joined Helen, a woman from England. Together they partnered with two Nepalese students. The four of them lived in a small village south of Katmandu and worked hard to improve lives there. The four of them taught English and created out-of-school activities for the children.

Brenin had been gone since late December. I read each of his letters with pride and felt the heart of my son shining into his community as he befriended the children and the elders. He referred to his Nepalese mother fondly as Ayma, which is Nepalese for "mother."

Shortly after April 1, I called the Student Partnership Program headquarters in London and told them I needed to speak with Brenin. We were finally able to arrange a time for him to call me from the only public phone, several miles down the road in the next village. It was evening in Nepal, and early morning in Traverse City. Over a crackling connection across thousands of miles, I told Brenin about Greg's diagnosis and didn't try to hide my sadness. I could hear the disbelief in his voice. He paused as his feelings choked in his throat. He asked, "Mom, what should I do?" We agreed to keep in touch, and I promised to call him if I needed him to come home.

I knew he was immersed in a once-in-a-lifetime experience, and that he wanted to finish the program, but three weeks later I reluctantly asked him to come back. I had reached a tipping point, I was losing my ability to manage all the demands of our life. Brenin would be such a help to us, caring for Emerson. He was the one person I could lean on.

Still, I hated to do it. He would have to break his commitment to the program and travel alone through Nepal. I read about the bloodshed of the Nepalese civil war and how civilians were caught in the crossfire. Brenin had confided to me how strongly Americans were disliked, and how he began to tell people he was from Canada.

But he immediately agreed to return. I knew it would take miles and weeks for him to appear. I was unable to sleep, watching the golden orb of the full moon setting in the west and imagining him working his way back to us.

16.

THE FIRST INGREDIENT

KATHERINE

I HAVE KEPT A GARDEN FOR THE PAST 30 YEARS. Even during the demanding days of medical school, in my rented house in inner-city Miami, the small triangular-shaped lot in the shadow of the concrete expressway arc called out for a garden. The relatively minuscule connection of tending to the lives of plants kept me grounded during the whirlwind of lectures and time in the hospital.

When we started driving back and forth to Ann Arbor and our days became filled with issues of life and death, we abandoned our gardens at home. They became choked with weeds, hiding flowers that had bloomed and died. I had created the beautiful landscape with exuberance, and now it defied me. The gardens were one more responsibility, a burden to us, especially Greg. He loved the colors of the flowers, marveled at the milkweed's lure of the monarch, and chuckled at the way the berries on the mountain ash quickly disappeared, devoured by a flock of cedar waxwings. But he resented the tether they placed on our free time. He pleaded with me to go for a walk or a sunset boat ride around the lake. That was when he still had some energy left; now he could barely walk around the block.

In early June, the gardens were a mirror image of our life. Chaos and neglect surrounded them, yet I was comforted by their swaying greenness. I believed in their innate goodness. All they needed was just a little love and an intelligent hand to discriminate what to let grow and what to prune. It was so much like Greg's immune system.

His body was overwhelmed by chaos and destruction. How could he make sense of it all?

I knew the job of his immune system—with its legions of cells and antibodies—was to comb through his entire body and know self from non-self. It was designed to attack, destroy, and consume unwanted invaders. The intelligence of this system was next to miraculous. Yet I was painfully aware that radiation and chemotherapy injured this powerful ally.

I consoled myself with the knowledge that I had been giving Greg medicinal mushroom extracts at the beginning and end of each day. The extracts contained large molecules known as beta-glucans that enhanced immunity. Diagrams of their molecular structure resembled huge antennae with arms. In scientific words, the arms were "branching side chains" that attached themselves to the membranes of the white cells. Like a key in a lock, they turned them on. The white cells became natural killer cells and could directly attack the tumor. The macrophages (whose name literally means "big eaters") were better able to engulf foreign particles, including cancer cells, cellular debris and bacteria.

These mushroom compounds also stimulated the production of healthy cells in the bone marrow, which was critical while going through chemotherapy. Therapy would be postponed if their numbers fell too low. I was encouraged by the research reporting that patients taking the mushroom compounds, most notably maitake and coriolus, had improvement in symptoms, enhanced survival, and tumor regression. Could they be Greg's master gardener, helping him know what to do with his body's chaos? Could they activate his battered immune system?

As I stood in the garden that June morning, the Parker family pulled into our driveway and came to our rescue. They brought their love and time. Parker, a seasoned gardener, knew just what the "jungle" and my family needed. He set us to work while their youngest daughter, Molly, played with Emerson. Parker's wife, Barb, brought food to eat, a white stuffed bunny for Emerson, and time without a clock. We leaned against them that day. Greg rested inside while I worked outside. I felt rejuvenated as I sat beside them in the understory of the pines, separating perennials from weeds. We spoke from our hearts with both lightness and sobriety. We pushed our wheel barrels and carried bushel baskets overflowing with weeds to the compost pile. The plants responded, shining back at us reclaimed. I meditated on Greg's immune system and envisioned it equally triumphant.

MUSHROOMS AND CONVENTIONAL THERAPY

More than two dozen human studies of PSK have been reviewed by experts at the University of Texas MD Anderson Cancer Center. Almost all of these studies were done in Japan and focused on cancer of the esophagus, stomach, colon, or breast. Most of them found that people with cancer were helped by PSK. People who received PSK with other treatments, such as surgery, chemotherapy, or radiation therapy, generally experienced longer periods of time without disease and higher survival rates compared with patients who received only standard treatment. Side effects from PSK in these studies were very mild. Smaller studies have suggested PSK may not be as effective against liver cancer or leukemia.

In November 2012, the FDA approved two clinical trials using "turkey tail" (PSK) at Bastyr University with patients with breast and prostate cancer. See www.bastyr.edu—news/research.

FOUR WAYS MUSHROOMS FIGHT CANCER:

- Protecting healthy cells from becoming cancerous
- Enhancing the immune system's ability to seek out and destroy cancer cells
- Helping cells regain normal cell division
- Preventing cancer spread

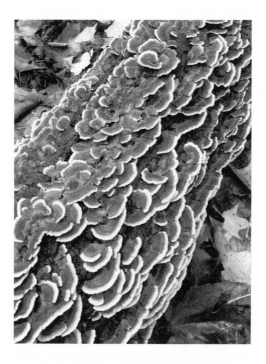

Turkey tail mushrooms.

MEDICINAL MUSHROOMS

The two most researched mushrooms for cancer support are maitake and Coriolus versicolor.

MAITAKE (GRIFOLA FONDOSA)

Maitake D-fraction is a specific component of the maitake mushroom that has been found to have a significant ability to stimulate the white blood cells especially the macrophages and killer T Cells. Further purification produces an even more potent version known as Maitake MD-fraction. It is found to be 30% more effective than the D-fraction. Both can be found in a liquid or capsule form.

- Dosage 0.5-1 mg per kg of body weight (35-70 mg) twice a day on empty stomach

CORIOLUS VERSICOLOR (AKA CLOUD FUNGUS MUSHROOM, TURKEY TAIL, YUN-ZHI)

PSK and PSP are closely related protein bound polysaccharides found in Coriollus versicolor. Like the compounds found in maitake, they enhance immune function.

- Dosage 3-6 grams per day in divided doses on empty stomach.

The research from Japan is based on mushrooms obtained from a hot water extraction rather than shredded mushrooms (biomass). It is more time intensive to produce, but ultimately researched to be more effective.

It is not necessary to take both maitake and PSK/PSP. They can be given in rotation, that is, one month of one and then one month of the other.

BRENIN ARRIVED IN THE U.S. IN MID-JUNE. His father dropped him off at our door, helped him with his backpack, and drove away with a small wave. Emerson watched from the window, then ran away to hide. She wouldn't come out for a half an hour, which was an eternity for her. I folded her brother into my arms and felt his warmth and his slightness. He never was a large person, but now he was taller and so much thinner. His eyes were a lighter blue and more penetrating, his cheekbones more pronounced with his leanness. He spoke more softly and moved more gently.

Brenin looked around his once familiar home and the spaciousness of the blue-green lake. Gone was the Nepalese village where twenty people could have lived in our contemporary home. His body was here but his mind drifted between worlds. I tried to see our world as he might. So much had changed since his departure eight months before. Greg was now critically ill and withdrawn, Emerson was older and more defiant, and Brenin's childhood dog, Free, had died.

I coaxed Emerson out from behind the couch. She'd known her brother once, but maybe not now. After all, he'd been gone almost a year. He produced gifts from his small bag. He had employed a tailor in the village to make a Nepalese outfit for her, a flowered smock that tied at the waist and loose pants. She smiled and ran to him.

Greg and Brenin had their own way. Brenin was very loyal to his father; Greg was the unwelcome stepfather. Greg loved Brenin from a distance, yet he was the one who had championed his education, his bedtime, and his work ethic. Greg could only parent through me, and we both hoped that one day his love would be reciprocated.

That night I dreamt that Brenin's "mother" in Nepal, his Ayma, was saying goodbye to him and to the sunshine he had brought to her family. I watched her go to him and place a mark on his forehead. She kissed him on each cheek. Then she turned away. Like me, like everyone I knew, all her losses rolled together into one. I wondered if she too had trouble feeling the depth of her sadness.

The dream swirled and turned into a huge tide pool. After moments of watching the powerful surging water, I took off my clothes and entered the pool. As I swam excitedly to the edge I could see everything. Surf was being created as water flowed into the pool from a larger nearby lake. For the first time in months, I awoke feeling full of life and adventure. I knew I was connected to something large and powerful.

THE NEXT DAY Greg went to the dentist at the oncologist's insistence. With the radiation and loss of protective saliva, his teeth were compromised, like so many things. The absence of saliva, a condition known as xerostomia, could lead to problems because it promoted tooth decay and gum disease. Mercifully, his dentist reported, "All is well." He mentioned in passing that he had had a dream about Greg and me. He didn't elaborate except to say that he knew we were going through a lot and that he was praying for us. I knew he was right; seen and unseen forces were with us.

I went to my office and met with Nancy and Sharon. Greg waited for me in the car; he was becoming too weak to walk or exercise. I heard the sobriety in their voices and saw the uncomfortable shifting of their eyes. I knew they could feel the magnitude of what I was going through, and saw Greg's death sitting on my shoulder.

We first discussed the easy details, such as how to share the after-hour calls. Then the conversation took a more serious turn as they told me how much they would pay to buy my share of the practice. I quickly calculated the figure in my head and realized that it was just enough to cover my overhead for the month. I was barely able to keep my finances afloat.

But that was how it was. I refused to dwell on what did not free me. I was tired of looking for love in these tokens of rejection. I was becoming a freer, truer warrior. I reminded myself that it was my choice to leave, and I entered that brighter truth as I closed the office door.

Greg and I drove across town to my potential new office on Front Street. I began to imagine a new reality as we strolled through the building and the neighborhood. It was a miracle to be so close to making an offer for the purchase of this old house! I was reminded of the dream of the surging water feeding into the pool and felt new energy entering into my life. The metaphor of my dream couldn't have been clearer.

IN THE DOCTOR'S LOUNGE at the hospital, I found a quiet corner and took a deep breath. I picked up the phone and called Dr. Tyler Curiel at Tulane University. Dr. Curiel was Andy Martin's physician and friend. To my complete disbelief, he answered the phone! I expected an answering machine or a secretary and had never dreamed he would answer the phone himself.

What prompted the call was Parker informing us last week that he had seen Andy on the *Today Show*. He was referring to the young medical student Greg had read about in the *Wall Street Journal* that distant day of April 1, 2004. It had been just nine weeks, yet it felt like a lifetime. When Parker mentioned this young man who was mysteriously linked to our path, I felt compelled to call Dr. Curiel.

And here he was, on the phone listening to my story about Greg. The first words out of his mouth were, "I am so sorry." The depth in his words spoke volumes. He, of all people, knew what we were up against. There was no need to explain our anguish or our fears.

He freely explained where he was in his work on this deadly cancer. He sounded cautiously excited and mentioned that he might be on the verge of a breakthrough. After months of dismal attempts, he and Andy were finally able to grow Andy's tumor cells in his laboratory. He explained how there were identifying markers on the cells that could lead to drugs that hadn't been tried before in treatment. He was sharing vital information with me, but with guarded optimism. I hung onto every word, knowing I was drawing hope from a shallow well. He advised us to continue with Greg's treatment, and offered to see him if things did not respond. He encouraged us "to stay the course and to keep in touch."

I was excited and tried to relay the conversation to Greg, but he was only vaguely interested. I mentioned Andy, but Greg refused to talk about him. It was too close. He simply said, "It's not helpful. It's not a good story."

Did Greg somehow know that Andy would die in a few short months? Could he foresee that, years later, in the wake of Hurricane Katrina, Dr. Curiel's cell research would almost be destroyed? Did he know that Dr. Curiel would ultimately abandon the field of sinus cancer research, never understanding how to halt its aggressiveness?

That day, however, I clung to Dr. Curiel's warm voice and his personal recommendations to us. "Go forward and contact me if the treatment is not successful. I will help reevaluate your husband with what I learn." It was something in the midst of so little.

Later that day, we drove back to the cottage and started the second half of Greg's treatment. It was frightening to watch him losing energy. He didn't want to go to the gym anymore or walk the dusty path around the lake. He was so exhausted that he started sleeping through the once terrifying radiation treatments. He could barely finish the whey shakes I made for him, and many ended up spilled in the back seat of the Subaru. I had long ago given up on the idea that he could swallow the pills of fish oil, amino acids, probiotics, and vitamins. Now I opened the capsules directly into the shake and hoped they would make it down his raging throat. I prayed over every item I gave to him: it was my first ingredient.

The rest of life was no simpler. Emerson became sick in the middle of the night with uncontrollable vomiting and diarrhea. My life felt like a battlefield as I was tending the people I loved. I thought of Walt Whitman, and how he moved through the Civil War encampments of injured soldiers, reading them lines of his poetry to ease their pain. I prayed that I could have his endurance and enlightened heart.

Brenin and I practiced yoga together every morning. It was a way to greet the day and bring structure to our lives. My body needed the stretching, but, more so, my mind needed the opportunity to focus on what was right in our lives.

Greg and I drove to his treatment and it felt good to be alone, just the two of us. When we arrived back at the cottage we discovered Greg's sisters, Laura and Amy, had come to play with Emerson. They were huddled together on the floor watching *The Little Mermaid*. Greg sat with them for a few moments, then he stood up and left the room. As he departed, he said, "It's all about a woman giving up her body to be with a man!" There was no pretending for him anymore.

Greg took me aside and told me I needed to be firmer with Emerson. I understood his request. He felt his energy lessening and he needed me to do the parenting for the two of us. Yet it seemed unreasonable while she was sick and I was fatigued and distracted. I sensed she needed the opposite of discipline. She needed to play and just let life flow.

I watched her cuddle and giggle with her Aunt Laura, a treasure to behold. Gently, I reminded myself that I was a good mother. In fact, I was a lovely mother. I just couldn't make some parts of this better; not for Emerson, for Greg, not for Brenin.

I couldn't change or control anything except my inner landscape. How could I do this? I closed my eyes and practiced the art of "tonglen," a meditation practice I'd learned years ago. It was a way to use the breath to move through the sticky parts of life. I closed my eyes and breathed in our struggle—the unfairness, the nightmare of ev-

eryone's suffering—Brenin's, Emerson's, Greg's, and mine. The difficulties felt like dark, smoky energy. With my breath, I moved them
into my chest, my lungs, my heart, and I held them there for a moment. Then I let my breath move to the back of my heart, into the
deepest and purest of places, where I found a lightness and vastness
that could hold it all. Then I breathed out surrender, acceptance,
and stillness. I sat like that for countless moments and worked with
my breath over and over again. I just let it be—all of it.

WE WATCHED A STORM BUILD IN THE DISTANCE and
move toward us across the lake. On the heels of the building wind,
a torrential downpour began. The moist winds suddenly released
all the hot tension in the summer air and replaced it with coolness
and rain. Rain was driving sideways across the deck and pounding
on the sliding glass door. Greg opened the door momentarily, and
the storm burst in on us with all its hurricane-like energy. A crazy idea came to him. He turned to us and asked, "Who wants to
stand in front of the door?" At first we hesitated, looking at him in
disbelief. Then Laura jumped up. Greg quickly slid the door open
and announced, " Here is your treatment!" Laura was anointed with
the blast of energized rain. The rest of us couldn't resist, and we
clamored for our turn as we lined up in front of Greg and the sliding door. Each blast invigorated and delighted us. Finally I gave a
"treatment" to dear Greg and we broke down and laughed at all the
absurdity and tragedy.

Later that night, I awoke suddenly from slumber, shaken. Sleep
would not come back to me, and I was alone. I crawled out of bed
and found a small light and my pen. I knew I needed to write, to
connect with the life we were living in all it rawness.

Sleep had eluded me for months. I recalled the nights in the beginning when I knew Greg was sick, but I didn't have a name for
it. I could barely relax beside him in the same bed because of his

labored breathing. I would lie there in the darkness, not daring to disturb his precious sleep. Now, months later, it was his pain that kept me awake. I found it impossible to sleep beside him. His pain frightened me and made me feel powerless.

I was equally frightened by the treatments. They had already taken so much life from him. How could he possibly endure the next three weeks? How much more could he take?

Greg confided something that captured what we both were thinking and feeling. "All of this would be so much easier if we knew it was working." But to go through the treatment and suffer terrific pain, become depleted, poisoned, and then…die? It was unbearable to think that this might be the outcome. Yet it was what we had to do.

Although we couldn't choose what would happen, we could choose our attitude. Against all odds, I visualized Greg surviving, and that he and I would continue to love one another and help others. I imagined Emerson returning to her school and her friends. We would begin to heal, rebuild, and cleanse. We would do this!

But the reality was that we had to go deeper still. Our faith in the unknown was all we had to lead us forward. I vowed to stay strong for all of us—for Greg, for Emerson, and for my own soul.

I lay in bed and cried, wishing I could have just one normal day, one day from our past when we were innocent and in love. A day when I could greet my husband, vital and alive with his wit and his smiling blue eyes. I would give everything for just such a day. I treasured our life, but had I treasured it enough? I vowed to stay awake to all that was right today. He was still here.

GREG BEGAN HIS FOURTH ROUND OF CHEMOTHERAPY, and Dr. Francisco was his usual professional self. If he did have any emotions, they were skillfully concealed from my scrutinizing eyes. As an oncologist, he saw many patients who smoked or drank heavily, and those were the obvious risk factors for cancers of the mouth, throat, and neck. Nearly transparent, Greg sat before him, a relatively young man who had lived a careful life; he'd never smoked, was a light drinker, exercised regularly, ate right, and kept his weight admirably low. He did all the things the cancer posters recommended to prevent the disease. Greg seemed to unnerve him, and I believed it was because he saw himself in Greg. He obviously had taken care of himself as well, and on most days believed he was protected—until he'd met Greg.

Greg didn't fit Franciso's model. He didn't have the familiar squamous cell cancer, he had the mysterious and rare SNUC. From the first day, I had the feeling that he felt truly sorry for Greg and would do his medical best. I also sensed that he believed Greg was a marked man, although he would never say that out loud.

As a doctor, as a man, as a person so similar to Greg, Dr. Francisco would not let himself get too close. He held us both at arm's length while Greg circled down the devastating spiral of chemotherapy and radiation. His own inner, pessimistic conviction would not stop his well-trained mind from trying to save Greg. He put his attention on the details of the treatment.

Once again, he voiced concerns about Greg's weight loss and lack of appetite. He took one look at his mouth, and didn't bother to lecture him to eat more. Instead, he prescribed Merinol, an oral form of marijuana containing inactive THC that he hoped would pick up Greg's appetite. I watched Greg fold the white prescription with a devil-may-care attitude. I looked down at the floor and held my tongue, concerned about his reaction to one more pill.

DR. ABDUL'S EXAM WAS MORE CONFRONTATIONAL. He scoped Greg's sinus and seemed frustrated when all he could see were secretions and "debris." His feeble attempts to be kind were limited by his inability to offer any comfort or hope.

I pressed him for useful information or suggestions—anything other than his silence and furrowed brow! He instructed Greg to begin nasal irrigation. Greg looked preoccupied, and I could tell that he was thinking about his dismal experience with the neti pot, and how nothing could get through the cancerous nostril. Dr. Abdul insisted that Greg take more nystatin for the sores and yeast infection that were torturing his mouth and tongue.

We spent several moments contemplating the benefits of another CAT scan to assess the effectiveness of the therapy so far. I was ambivalent; I knew that positive results from the scan might shorten the radiation treatment, but at the same time I was afraid the scan would confirm our worst fears and reveal the treatment was not working.

As we drove home together, Greg reminded me that the tumor was very evident two months ago when Dr. Abdul first examined him. Now all Dr. Abdul could see was snotty debris. Could it be that the tumor was in retreat—wasn't that what we wanted?

I remembered what Bob Leichtman said to me—that we would have to go for broke! We were at a place where we needed his body to flush, digest, and cleanse the stagnation. I needed to do more research!

LUMBROKINASE

This is a unique proteolytic enzyme derived from the earthworm and used for hundreds of years in Chinese Medicine. It is useful in hyper coagulation states (found in the majority of patients with cancer) and in situations with decreased blood flow. It is stronger than nattokinase, another proteolytic enzyme created from fermented soy protein. It does not interfere with the blood-clotting cascade and does not cause bleeding. It works primarily by lowering fibrin and fibrinogen. Elevated fibrinogen levels in the blood have been associated with increased risk of metastasis (spreading) of cancer.

- Recommended doses: 20 mg 1-3 times per day on an empty stomach

Research:

- (http://bloodjournal.hematologylibrary.org/content/96/10/3302.full
- http://www.nature.com/bjc/journal/v109/n5/full/bjc2013443a.html
- http://www.nutricology.com/infocus/pdfletters/InFocus_2009Mar_ Earthworms.pd)

GRAPE SEED EXTRACT

Grape seed extract (GSE) is a byproduct of the wine industry and it is produced from the grinding of the grape seed into an extract. It has recently been supported in clinical research as having anti-cancer properties. Specifically GSE has been shown in animal research to generate DNA damage in cancer cells and inhibit the cells ability to repair. Importantly, there is no associated toxicity to supplementation.

Recent research has focused on its usefulness in head and neck cancers and aggressive colon cancer.

- Greg took a supplement that contained 100 mg three times per day with his proteolytic enzymes. Some research suggests 150 mg per day.

Research:

- ww.naturalnews.com/034893_grape_seed_extract_cancer_cells_DNA. html#

- http://www.sciencedaily.com/releases/2013/01/130117105843.htm

- http://www.medicalnewstoday.com/articles/263332.php

GREG'S TUMOR MAY HAVE SHRUNK, but the thick, sluggish stuff was not a good thing either. The surface gunk was a symptom of an underlying pattern of inflammation and stagnation that involved Greg's entire circulatory system, including the lymph tissue and blood stream.

As a young medical student, I was taught how cancer patients are at an increased risk for unwanted blood clots. The "stickier" blood makes a person three to five times more likely to develop recurrent clots and life-threatening pulmonary emboli (a blood clot blocking an artery leading to the lung).

This propensity to clot or coagulate has other serious implications; the imbalance fuels the growth and the spread of cancer, known as metastasis. This happens because cancer cells release a chemical to ensure their ultimate survival. The chemical, called a pro-coagulant, activates platelets (blood particles involved in clotting) and speeds up their making of a protein called fibrin, which knits other blood proteins together. These proteins, now all close and sticky, make the blood more prone to clot.

Soon the activated platelets gather around the tumor and shield it from the body's immune response and its natural killer cells. Furthermore, these same hijacked platelets build paths from the cancerous tumor into the nearby bloodstream, allowing the cancer to spread to distant sites. The activated platelets stimulate the growth of blood vessels (angiogenesis) that feed the cancer cells and help them grow even more.

How could I stop the platelets from activating? It was not as easy as Dr. Abdul suggested. Salt-water rinses alone would not wash the problem away. I researched ways to give Greg phytochemicals (chemicals made from plants) that would block the activation of the platelets and work as natural blood thinners. Big on the list were proteolytic enzymes; substances that break down proteins, like fibrin and procoagulants. Perhaps the best-known proteolytic enzyme is bromelain, which is derived from pineapples. Plastic surgeons tell their patients to eat lots of pineapple before and after surgery to reduce bruising and faster recovery.

I tested Greg's tendency for hypercoagulation that day, and his levels came back slightly elevated. I started giving him capsules of concentrated bromelain three times a day, along with other enzymes. The one enzyme that gave me real hope was serratia peptidase, from the intestine of the silk worm. It allows the emerging moth to dissolve its cocoon. Scientists had found a merciful way to produce the enzyme—without having to harvest and kill the silk worm—from the bacteria, serratia bacterium. It is regarded by practitioners in Asia and Europe as the most powerful of the proteolytic enzymes. I was excited by its long history of use in sinusitis and respiratory infections. It seemed like the perfect choice for Greg.

I calculated the amount of proteolytic proteins that Greg would need to take—not one tablet, but five tablets three times a day, and on an empty stomach! I combined the enzymes tablets with other potent plant extracts which included green tea (EGCG), that would block vascular endothelial growth factor (VEGF) stimulating his blood vessels; curcumin, with its NFkB reducing ability (the master switch for inflammation); and grape seed extract, which among other things, interferes with the platelets clustering together. I believed that Greg and his phyto-cocktails would be stronger than his tumor.

LIFE KEPT INTERJECTING ADDITIONAL COMPLICATIONS. We returned to Ann Arbor for a week of treatment, which included his last two rounds of chemotherapy, along with five daily doses of radiation. We soon discovered we'd left his prescriptions and supplements behind in Traverse City. This meant I had to scurry about, trying to renew our provisions instead of holding Greg's hand.

As I trudged into the co-op to purchase vanilla whey (which, as it turned out, he hated), I wondered, "How is it that I am making a terrible thing even worse?" When I went to pick up Emerson and Brenin from the library, I realized I'd lost my parking stub, which I needed to exit the parking deck. Brenin was visibly frustrated as I fumbled about, looking for it in my purse. He wanted to be on time to pick up Greg from the hospital. It felt like all my best laid plans were unraveling.

Greg's radiation treatments were at a different time each day, so there was really no planning or efficiency in our life. On the second day there was a small window of opportunity for us to be together between his chemotherapy and radiation, and we went to get some lunch. My beeper kept going off while we were trying to eat. The office was calling me with some patient messages, and I was also trying to arrange for a neighbor to pick up my office paperwork and bring it to me when we returned home. Fortunately for Greg, the cell phone died and I was required to set off in search of a pay phone. As I walked the busy street, my mind calmed down and I stepped away from the chaos.

All the distraction and bullshit tried my patience and irritated Greg. He was struggling to stay alive, and all the juggling and multitasking was making me crazy. Greg wanted us to slow down; he could no longer tolerate living in a fast-paced world. He deserved this, and I vowed once again to set our compass toward a simpler way. He had become a great teacher to me. Why was this so incredibly hard? Where was the peace that could embrace even this? I needed to step beyond my desire to control life.

That evening we all sat down to watch the movie *The Big Fish*. The big fish was big because it didn't get caught—by fear, temptation, or even death. It was priceless to hear Greg laughing and enjoying himself. Our love was strong and unique like the love between the man and woman in the movie. I felt my kindred connection to the man's wife as she climbed without hesitation into the bath, fully dressed, to be with the dying man she adored. With each heart-wrenching day, I knew I was more completely in love with Greg, and the movie inspired me to become even more generous, accepting, and unconditional.

Still, I continued to feel disappointed when I offered him food, drinks, and supplements that he struggled with or rejected outright. But something had changed in me. As the days wore on, I didn't feel personal rejection anymore. I kept patiently offering what I believed he needed. It was good for him to express his will and decide what he could or couldn't tolerate of my offers. He had no choice about the pain that filled his world.

PROTEOLYTIC ENZYMES

These have many important anticancer effects. They increase the production of cancer blocking anti-proteases, inhibit angiogenesis and metastasis, enhance the immune response, and promote differentiation of cancer cells.

Clinical studies suggest that proteolytic enzymes improve the general condition of patients and their quality of life and produce slight to modest increase in life expectancy. Reference Drugs 2000;59:769-80.

Recent research has shown that these enzymes are absorbed intact across the GI membrane. Previously they were thought to be broken down by digestion.

Two caveats to get the most from these enzymes are to use a quality product and to take an adequate dosage. If potency is not listed, best to avoid. Also use combinations of enzymes (similar to the mixture used in the clinical studies such as Wobezyme or Zymactive) rather than any single enzyme.

Dosages

- Pancreatin 300-900 mg 3 times a day
- Chemotrypsin 180-540 mg 3 times a day
- Trypsin 3-9 mg 3 times a day
- Bromelain 250-750 mg 3 times a day
- Papain 50-150 mg 3 times a day
- Serratia peptidase 50-150 mg 3 times a day

Avoid use 2-3 days prior to surgery as it may increase risk of bleeding, However, after surgery, they are important and may protect from swelling and lymphedema. (See Lumbrokinase on page 217.)

If allergic to pork avoid pancreatic enzymes. If allergic to pineapple, avoid bromelain. If allergic to papaya, avoid papain.

17.
MI SHEBERAKH

GREG

ON FRIDAY, JIM AND SHELLEY arrived at the cottage to take me to my last chemotherapy treatment. I was frightened, but they gently nudged me into their car and encouraged me to focus on the fact that it would be over soon.

We parked the car, navigated our way through the halls of the Cancer Center, and ultimately made our way to the chemo lounge. We walked past the private room where Katherine and I had made defiant love in the face of the enemy. Now two great friends, my chosen family, were holding me up across the finish line.

The three of us had become fast friends many years ago, almost as soon as we met. Shelley and I found each other as graduate students when she volunteered to help with the research project I was conducting for my dissertation. She was a tall and slender woman with thick, curly black hair. She impressed me as a bright, insightful person with a magnetic intensity. She was quick-witted, and we enjoyed laughing together at the absurdities of life.

Shelley was unfailingly generous, but her greatest gift to me by far was the introduction to her husband, Jim. She had "a feeling" we would like each other, and it was clear from the first moment that her intuition was right. Jim didn't need to warm up to people; he was born warmed up. He was naturally kind and keenly tuned into the needs of others. A nurturing soul, Jim was the kind of man you would describe as "being in touch with his feminine side." He was always up for an adventure, and over the years we had certainly found our share of them.

Shelley often had "a feeling" about things, and she didn't hesitate to share her intuitions. She told me shortly after my diagnosis that she "had a feeling" that I was going to be "okay" and that I was going to beat the cancer.

Shelley and Jim pulled chairs up next to my recliner and clasped my hand as the chemo nurse positioned the transparent bags. The nurse tried to find one remaining vein that could receive an IV needle. That day my right arm was a no-go. The nurse tried to work her way around my needle phobia by choosing a smaller diameter needle used with children. She inserted it into a vein on the top of my left hand, bypassing my skinny left arm, which had developed large, purplish bruises from the earlier injections.

I closed my eyes as I felt the promised "poke" and I squeezed Jim's hand as the chemo began to rush through my vein. I tried to focus on his strength and energy rather than the needle and the drugs. Shelley began to sing *Mi Sheberakh*, a traditional Jewish prayer for the sick. It was overwhelming, and I broke down and wept. I had reached the end of a long and painful journey that had destroyed me. There was nothing left. I knew right then that I was going to die.

The chemo nurse returned and slowly withdrew the IV. "There you go," she said. "Are you okay?" I didn't answer. What could I say? It was obvious to anyone that I wasn't. She continued, "Just take all the time you need before you get up." What else could she say? A little bit of extra recliner time was all that remained on the schedule.

I sat motionless for what seemed like a long time. I could say that I was busy collecting my thoughts, but that would be a lie. Collecting my thoughts was impossible. Most of them had deserted me a long time ago, and what little remained of my mind had shattered into pieces. The combination of the chemo, radiation, and cancer had defeated me. I was a broken man.

Shelley and Jim helped me from the recliner and held each of my arms as we wound down the row of recliners and back through the lounge. The two nurses at the nurses' station paused momentarily from their flurry of activity to say good-bye. Neither of them said "good luck." I felt as though the nurses were paying their last respects as Jim and Shelley ushered me past their station in a funeral-like procession.

BACK AT THE COTTAGE, Shelley returned to Lansing, and Jim and I decided to buy some fireworks to celebrate the end of my treatment. I was exhausted, but I was determined to go. We decided to drive across the state line to Toledo and buy "real fireworks"—the kind that were illegal in Michigan. I rationalized the trip. All I had to do was sit in the car while Jim drove. Right? Katherine questioned whether it was "good for me" to run around and do things with Jim when I was so sick. Rather than depleting my energy, Jim was like the Energizer Bunny, with vitality to spare. With so much pep, I thought, he could recharge me.

My fascination with firecrackers and fireworks began when I was a young boy. My mother had an explosion of her own when she discovered the box full of cherry bombs and M-80s that I'd bought through the mail. They were powerful, dangerous, and illegal—the perfect combination that made them so exciting!

We climbed into Jim's new Highlander and headed south toward the state line. I'd heard several cautionary stories from others of past attempts to purchase the forbidden fireworks. But Jim and I had a foolproof plan. We would grab the goods, hide the contraband under several blankets, and drive carefully to avoid a traffic violation.

We made our way across the border into the Buckeye state and pulled off the interstate. I assumed we would be greeted by an abundance of stores and roadside stands offering fireworks for sale. I was wrong. Instead we were met by the same mishmash of gas stations, drug stores, and junky strip malls that infected the rest of America. Where were all the fireworks? We decided to pull into what looked like a family-style restaurant and ask the locals for inside advice. A young man seated by himself was quite amused when we told him about our clandestine mission. "Well," he said, "I always get mine in Michigan."

"Michigan?"

"Yup," he said, between mouthfuls of mashed potatoes. "Michigan. There's stores right along the freeway, across the border."

Sure enough, we found the stores exactly as he had described. It was embarrassing because they were hard to miss, with huge, colorful signs in front of them that screamed "FIREWORKS." Like so many things in life, the obvious remained invisible from our prejudiced view.

Jim and I made our way into a huge pole barn crammed with an abundance of rockets and shells. A young, tattooed man who smelled like cigarettes rushed over to greet us. I made it clear up front that we wanted to get "real" fireworks, not some wimpy-ass sparklers or little snakes that crawl out of a black pellet. *Real* fireworks!

The salesman flashed a smile as wide as his thin face. He had the same look of amusement as the man in the restaurant. He quickly assured us that his fireworks were, in fact, the "real deal." When we asked how he could sell illegal fireworks in Michigan, he was quick to give us a lawyer-like loophole explanation: You could buy fireworks in Michigan, you just couldn't shoot them off.

We filled the Highlander to the brim with the long, colorful packages and headed back to Sue's cottage. The return drive seemed much longer. Dark thoughts plagued me. I wondered if I would live long enough to see the blasts of color explode in the dark sky over our lake that Independence Day.

By then I'd spent a lot of time thinking about my impending death, and fireworks figured in my thoughts. I knew I wanted to be cremated, and I wanted my cremains to be mixed with gunpowder, packed into big shells, and fired into the sky over Lake Michigan.

Jim dropped me off at the Silver Lake cottage and headed home with the fireworks payload. I fell on the couch. I knew Katherine would worry about my exhaustion and pain; I obsessed about it myself all the time. However, an adventure with Jim was one of the few things left in my life to look forward to, and I wasn't about to give it up.

KATHERINE

I RETURNED HOME LATE THAT NIGHT and immediately felt the gravity of the situation as I entered the dim and silent house. Kate and Mike had driven Greg back to Traverse City after his radiation treatment. He was stretched out on the sofa, motionless, and our friends sat beside him in the nearby chairs. These were friends who always knew what to do, but now they sat with their hands folded. Their eyes met mine with all the seriousness of the moment. Without words I knew the day had been difficult and they felt powerless to help Greg. I entered their silence.

I looked down at Greg and felt that some terrible trick had been played on him. He had aged several decades in just a few short weeks. His once thick, chestnut hair was now just wisps of white. His warm and twinkling blue eyes, now absent of eyelashes, were red-rimmed and dull grey. His clothes swallowed up his skeleton-like frame. How did all this happen without me fully registering it? Where was the man I knew?

He looked up at me and his cracked lips forced a smile. He patted the couch for a moment, then changed his mind and closed his eyes. I stood paralyzed, at a loss for what to do. Then I realized I had to step through my sadness and despair. He was up to his neck in quicksand and sliding deeper each moment. He didn't need any more empathy—it only amplified what he already felt.

How terrible had it become? His energy was so low and his pain so immense that he couldn't speak. He could barely open his mouth. It was impossible for him to eat solid food and he struggled to simply swallow a mouthful of liquid. He was critical of everything. I let his irritability and sullen mood slide past me, knowing I had become the only safe place for him to express the pain he carried. I was happy to take whatever negative energy he could release. Without judgment.

That night I needed to be the person that he had been for so many. For years, I'd watched him effortlessly provide encouragement to countless others—and to me. It was what had drawn me to his side and won my heart. His spirit was generous and bright and could coax even the most taciturn and skeptical person into conversation. There were so few barriers for Greg; nothing was impossible.

So what was stopping me? What were my barriers—fear, doubt, some sense of smallness? I stepped through them. I prayed for his life and our love. I visualized Greg in all his perfection and his basic goodness. This was what I held onto as I tended to his temporary state of disease and pain. I brought cool compresses to his forehead and rubbed his feet. I just kept holding on, choosing love over fear.

GREG

THE PAIN IN MY MOUTH, ONCE CONFINED to swallowing, intensified and became a deep throbbing ache that was unrelenting. I couldn't sleep. I was twisting and turning, buffeted by wave after wave of sharp, shocking pain. Finally I couldn't stand it anymore, and I begged Katherine to take me to the emergency room. I needed something to put me out of my misery. I didn't want to start taking narcotics, but I saw no choice.

I had put off going to the emergency room for as long as I possibly could. I was afraid that if I were admitted, I would never make it back out alive. My earlier premonition that I would die in the same hospital bed as my friend, Marilyn, was coming closer and closer to reality.

KATHERINE

GREG AWOKE IN THE EARLY HOURS of the morning and insistently shook my shoulder. He was ready to go into the hospital. We dressed quickly and stepped out into the moist air of the early morning. It felt good to be moving toward the help he needed.

We drove to town as the sun was rising, and met the resident on call for oncology patients in the hospital. I was relieved by her kindness and attentiveness to Greg. She surmised that his pain was from mucositis, the inevitable destruction of the skin lining the mouth and digestive tract. As she listened to our story, she gave Greg the long overdue praise that he so deserved. She pointed out that most people would have been on more pain medicine, much earlier, including both short- and long-acting narcotics.

She wrote prescriptions for Duragesic capsules and lidocaine swishes to rinse in his mouth and provide anesthesia to the tortured nerve endings of his lips and tongue. She noticed that he had lost some weight, but assured him the need for the feeding tube was behind him. As we left the clinic that morning, nothing had really changed, yet we felt transformed. Someone had finally heard us and witnessed our suffering. The young doctor offered him some respite, some response besides surrender. I prayed for the medicine to help.

Greg fell asleep as soon as we returned to the cottage. He woke up several hours later and immediately encouraged me to call Randy, a friend of ours who was a surveyor. "You'll need a survey of the Front Street property if you want to buy it," he said through his barely moving lips, a sign his life was flowing again.

AFTER DINNER Jim, our architect, called and asked how things were going. I had consulted with him about the Front Street house when I first became serious about it. He'd met with the city's zoning and coding departments about converting the old house into a medical office and told me we only had to build a barrier-free bathroom and clarify the parking lot plan. Could it really be that easy? Was it really going to happen?

My mind raced with questions about hiring employees, purchasing equipment, and creating patient charts. When would I want to open the office? When would I be able? I stopped and took a breath. *Flow.* Greg suggested I create a timeline to help steady my mind. I would do anything—a timeline, or whatever—I just wanted to hang onto the unrealistic belief that it could direct the flow of time and assure me of what it would bring.

The next morning I drove into town to meet the Jim. There was still dew on the grass, glistening in the early morning sunlight. Soon Jim drove up and parked under the old, defiant maple tree that stretched upward 30 feet, holding its place in a sea of asphalt. He stepped out of his car with blueprints under his arm. I knew they were a draft of his vision, and he appeared eager to share them.

I was overcome by the magnitude of what I had to do—give birth to something that had intimidated me for so many years. In that moment, my guard was down. Maybe it was the sweetness of the early June morning or the way Jim won my trust, but my pretense was gone. There was no place to hide as tears gathered in my eyes and spilled down my cheeks. I confessed to him what I was fighting desperately to hold back. "I don't think I can go forward with this. Greg needs me. I'm afraid he's going to die and I don't think I can do this without him!"

He reached out and hugged me. After what seemed like an eternity he asked, "What will you do then?" He neither denied my reality nor collapsed into it. I looked up at him with his head haloed by the stubborn maple and its bounty of leaves. I knew what I had to do. I needed to go forward with my dream, even with all the tender and terrible truth surrounding me. There was no place else to go other than this small stepping forward into the promise of tomorrow.

I looked into Jim's kind eyes and said, "Let's see your design." The office, my practice, insisted on being born.

THE DURAGESIC PATCH turned out not to be the panacea we were hoping for. Greg's pain was unshakable. It sat front and center in our lives, dictating our every move. Despite my inquiries, Greg could not begin to describe how hard everything was for him, and he stopped trying. He refused to talk about the medicine, his pain, his cancer. He kept a wide margin from Emerson and me, as he needed more space to cope and attempt to survive. To my surprise, Emerson skipped right through the land mines and "No Trespassing" signs Greg erected. She alone could find the way to make the most joyful, gentle contact. Intuitively she knew the spaces on Greg's body where his defenses were down—his fingers, his arm, the soft spot on his belly. And then their love dance would begin. Her ability to find the openings despite his grimaces never ceased to amaze me.

Thankfully, we were on the home stretch of the radiation treatments. We had been told that they would occur over eight weeks, but never the exact number. Now as we rounded into the final days we learned that the magic number was 35. We were perched at number 31 and could perform the final countdown on one hand. The last treatment would be on Thursday, July 1. Despite the horrific nature of those remaining few days, a slight hint of euphoria began to infuse the air.

I thought of how Greg loved numbers and counting. When he was a small boy, he lived within a short bicycle ride to a nearby gas station. He started to collect bottle caps in order to gain entrance to a live children's broadcast of "Buckaroo Rodeo" on the local television station. He cleverly devised a way to rescue discarded caps out of the soft drink machine at the gas station with the assistance of a simple magnet tied to the end of an old string. He succeeded in acquiring all the bottle caps he needed, and won a coveted spot on the show.

Counting seemed to steady him, and allowed him to accomplish things that most people would never be able to do. He called it his "chunk it theory." Just one thing at a time: back then it was a bottle cap, now it was a radiation treatment. Anything was possible if you broke it down into small pieces and tackled them one at a time.

As I thought back over the seemingly endless trips to the Cancer Center, I wished I had remembered that story. I would have bought Greg 35 colorful marbles. He could have dropped one marble into a big glass jar after each radiation treatment. Today he would have just four marbles left before him, waiting to be dropped into the sea of others.

I savored this light-hearted image because my medical mind was well aware that the effects of radiation were exponential in nature. As the treatments progressed, each one became increasingly important, and destructive. The vivid image of the marbles and the large jar filled with colorful spheres of glass lingered in my mind, like an altar of tribute to my tenacious husband.

ON DAY 32 OF GREG'S RADIATION, I made a radical move. I spent a day working in the office of an internist, Dr. Jack Johnson.

We had corresponded for several months—an accountant who helped him develop the framework for his new practice had given me his name and suggested I call him—yet we hadn't met.

Jack had something that eluded me. It wasn't a degree, a certificate, or even a lucrative salary—it was his independence. Like me, he had been a partner with fellow physicians in a large medical group. But he wanted something different. He escaped the rat race with insurance companies and developed a model where he could spend more time with his patients. He simply exchanged his knowledge, compassion, and time for money. Straight up. He set the rules fairly. He had actually done what I only dreamed of doing. I had to go to his office and see for myself.

And so, of all improbable moments, I went to East Lansing to spend the afternoon with him. Brenin assured me that he would take care of Emerson and drive Greg to his appointment at the Cancer Center. As I drove away that day, I reassured myself that everyone would survive my absence.

Dr. Johnson's office was located in a professional building along the banks of the Red Cedar River. As I pulled up in my car and turned off the engine, I could hear the distant murmur of water flowing. I gathered myself together, clasped a small notebook, and walked into the building, prepared to meet my fellow traveler.

I entered the office and was surprised by how unremarkable it was; it looked just like any other medical office in the country. The small waiting room was comfortably decorated with upright, cloth-covered chairs and a corner table. A half wall separated the room, and a receptionist sat behind it, talking quietly on the phone. She hung up and warmly greeted me. Dr. Johnson was just as welcoming. He knew no details of my personal life or what it had taken for me to carve out the few hours we would spend together.

He looked much as I had imagined with graying hair at his temples, kind eyes, and a stethoscope draped around his neck. He was professionally dressed in a white shirt, no tie, and black trousers. He ushered me past several exam rooms, into the inner sanctum of his private office. As we talked, he explained how he had chosen to make this bold step—dissolving his contracts with insurance companies and the large group practice. The fast pace and the tyranny of it all had brought him to a crossroad. He needed to either stop practicing medicine altogether or find a new way to do it. Doing the same old thing was killing him. I sensed that he wasn't using euphemisms.

I spent the day with him, sitting in on all of his patient encounters. He would do his traditional examination in one room, then invite the person into his office lined with medical textbooks and a wide wooden desk. He sat across from them and discussed his diagnosis and treatment recommendations. His medical records were no more complicated than a fountain pen and a piece of paper.

I learned all sorts of medical details, but what I really savored was the contrast between us. Here was a man at ease with himself and his choosing; he was a free man. There was an intimacy and honesty in that truth.

I knew that I, too, could be my own person. I would just have to follow my husband's mantra and "chunk it." I would take one step after the other and discover my own way of doing the work that I loved. I wasn't going to follow the specific path of Dr. Johnson: he did it his way, my path was different. It was not just the structure of the delivery system with insurance companies, but also the content of what I wanted to offer and the nuances of the process. I thought of the quote by Joseph Campbell:

"If you can see your path laid out in front of you step by step, you know it's not your path. Your own path you make with every step you take. That's why it's your path."

BY THE TIME I GOT BACK TO THE SILVER LAKE COTTAGE, it was 7 p.m. I knew it was late. Brenin came out to the car to greet me, and warn me. In three sentences he brought me up to speed. We didn't have enough vegetables for dinner, Emerson was hungry, and Greg, because of his exhaustion and pain, was unable to play with her so Brenin could cook. My confidence had followed me home that night. I hugged him and told him everyone was going to be all right. Soon Emerson was on my lap eating fresh blueberries, Brenin was making do with the ingredients we did have, and Greg listened as I shared the life I had discovered in four short hours. Brenin conceded that he had battled Greg to the end in a game of Risk—and lost. We all breathed a sigh of relief. Our family had survived another day.

That night Greg woke up and told me he felt cared for and loved. His skin felt better, and he thought maybe the lotion that I rubbed on him nightly might be helping. This small acknowledgement meant so much to me; it gave me the encouragement I needed to keep going. It seemed I had discovered my own servant's heart.

SKIN LOTION

Take care to avoid too much soap when bathing as it is dries out the skin. Hot water can also be drying.

A combination of herbs including calundula, aloe vera and hyaluronic acid has been found to be helpful in the care of skin during radiation.

Other good lotions include emu oil, shea butter, avocado, astathaxin, and Vitamin E.

18.

THE LAST MARBLE

GREG

THE DOORS IN THE RECEPTION AREA of the radiation clinic swung wide open and a tech came out to escort me to my last blast of radiation. We walked at a snail's pace on the well-worn path past the nursing station and down the windowless hall. I walked into the dressing room where a small group of men waited wordlessly to be taken to one of the treatment rooms. At the starting point of their treatment, they appeared healthy; unlike me, they still had some good meat on their bones.

The scene in the locker room seemed like a perfect picture of what people looked like "before" and "after" cancer treatment. I had recently come across a "before" picture of Katherine and myself that we'd taken in a photo booth at the Honolulu airport. We were tan, happy, and in love, wearing plumeria leis around our necks. I cried when I found the photograph. Everything but the love was gone.

I went through the usual routine of stripping off my clothes. It was no longer necessary to fuss with unbuckling my belt and unzipping my jeans. I had lost so much weight that my pants fell off if I didn't hook one of my thumbs though a front belt loop as I walked. I had given up trying to tie the gown in the back and simply tied it in the front. I never did have the patience to fumble around with it, and now I didn't have the energy either.

The tech took me back to one of the treatment rooms. I saw a red warning light flashing above the door and saw a sign that a treatment session was still in progress. We waited for a few minutes until the light stopped flashing. Mary and another technician came out of the control room and entered the treatment room to help the patient off the table and back to the dressing room. She gave me a thumb's up as she walked by and promised that she would come right back.

The radiation machine was waiting for me as always. It took quite a bit of time and considerable effort for me to climb up on the table. The technician grabbed a long pole and squinted his eyes as he surveyed the dozens of green masks on the wall. "I think this is yours," he muttered, more to himself than to me, as he snagged one of the nylon masks with the pole. It was mine all right. On a small white stripe were the bold black letters GREGORY HOLMES, 11/28/52. The only thing missing was the date of my death.

Mary, the friendly tech, floated into the room like an apparition, approached the table, and immediately grabbed my hand. "You made it!" she exclaimed. "It's your last treatment!"

"Yup," I said, blinking my eyes in a futile effort to hold back my tears. I peered though the two small eyeholes in my mask at Mary. Her eyes were wet also.

"I got you a little something from the gift shop—to celebrate," she said. "I'll give it to you in a few minutes, when we're done."

She squeezed my hand, promised once again that she would be right back, and left the room with the male tech. There was a loud clank as the door bolted behind them, and the warning buzzer sounded to announce that treatment was about to begin.

The room darkened and the machine came to life, emitting a whirring noise. Mary's voice came softly through the loudspeakers. "Greg, we're starting now." I looked up and saw Mary sitting in the driver's seat at the control board. Floating above her head was a bright blue balloon. I gulped back more tears, limply raised my right hand, and gave her my last thumb's up.

That treatment session seemed to end before it began. I was so eager to leave the Center and be done with the whole damn thing. Mary and the male tech came into the room. Mary held a big blue balloon that had "HAPPY BIRTHDAY!!" written on it in glittery silver letters. "I'm sorry," she said, turning red with embarrassment, "but they didn't have one that said, 'Congratulations!'" Mary was just like all the other generous people that I had met in my life; they always apologized that they hadn't done more.

I quickly attempted to rescue her from embarrassment by thanking her for her gift and reminding her that there was no need. It's the kind of awkward thing you say to someone so they don't feel so awkward.

The male technician approached me with my green mask in his hand and asked me if I wanted to take it home with me. I turned and looked at him with disbelief. What the hell would I do with it? Hang it on the wall as a souvenir? "Just burn it," I replied. There was no way I wanted to remember the torture I had endured.

Mary took me by the arm in an attempt to steady me as I teetered down the hallway to the men's dressing room. She waited patiently outside while I fumbled about, trying to undo my gown and put my oversized jeans back on.

I thanked her again for all that she had done during my treatment, and, in keeping with her character, she replied that she "really didn't do anything." I was dumfounded. She was the only person at the Center who really seemed to care about me.

We hugged each other and said our final goodbyes. She passed the balloon to me as if she were giving me my diploma. "You did it!" she called out as I stumbled through the doors into Katherine's arms.

I did it all right. I wasn't going to die in the hospital after all. I was going home.

WHEN WE RETURNED to the cottage I crumpled onto the couch and watched everyone else clean up the cottage and prepare to go back home to Traverse City. I always prided myself on being an efficient and fruitful person, but the cancer took both of those qualities away from me. I could tell you that I felt useless, and that would be true, but actually it was worse than that. I felt like a burden to everyone, especially Katherine. She would never admit it, and she never said or did anything that would suggest that she felt that way. Yet it's a fact that a person with a malady, even the flu, is a burden. Illness interferes with your life and the lives of others. As I watched Katherine and my sisters carry our suitcases and unused groceries to the car, I felt guilty about the real load they were carrying.

Outside by the car I spied Luke across the dirt road fussing with his white van. I crossed the street and climbed up the rutted dirt driveway. The yard was cluttered with the usual assortment of rusting bikes and abandoned toys. Luke stared, and I gave him a wave and called out to him in an effort to let him know that I was coming with peaceful intentions. I wondered if any neighbors on the lake ever stopped at his house for a non-complaining type of visit.

"Luke," I started, "I want you to know I'm done with my treatment and that we're going home now."

Luke looked at me with a knitted brow. His hardened, deeply lined face was like a closed book that hadn't been read for many years. "You comin' back this way?" he finally asked.

"Nope," I replied. "There's nothin' more they can do for me."

"You're gonna' be all right," Luke said firmly, pointing at me with his wrench for emphasis. I was surprised and pleased to hear his prophecy.

"I just want to thank you for being a good neighbor and helping us keep an eye on things, like the lawn," I said. "That really helped."

He tilted his head down and kicked the dirt with his worn-out work boot. True, he probably never was a man of many words, but at that instant he was caught totally off guard and didn't know what to say. I would bet a million dollars that no one before had called him a good neighbor.

We said our awkward goodbyes and I climbed into Flow. I stuck my hand out her window and waved to Luke as we pulled away. He raised his wrench in response; he and the lake disappeared from the rear view mirror.

KATHERINE

WE HAD ONE LAST APPOINTMENT before the ordeal was complete. On the way out of town, we stopped to meet with Dr. Abdul. The clinic visit was shorter than usual, and perfunctory; no new ground was covered. Dr. Abdul seemed preoccupied, and I wondered if he was thinking about another difficult case. Or was it his way of protecting himself from any feelings he might have as we said our goodbyes? I felt the river of patients that preceded us and would, just as certainly, flow behind us. Greg reached out, took both of Dr. Abdul's hands, and said, "Thank you for all you have done for me. I know you did your best and I am grateful for that."

Dr. Abdul quickly stepped back from him and looked away from Greg's tearful eyes. "You don't need to thank me. I was only doing my job," he said brusquely. And that was how we ended our relationship with Dr. Abdul.

We packed up our tent as the last marble entered the jar.

PART TWO

"Life shrinks or expands in proportion to one's courage"–Anais Nin

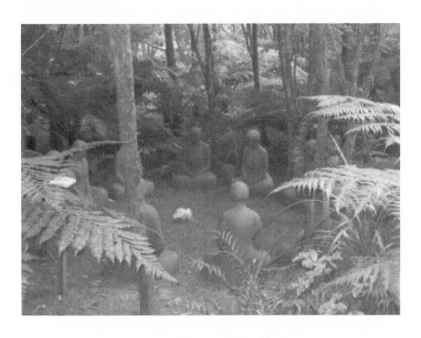

Bronze statues in the New Zealand bush 2/25/04.

19.

A CIRCLE OF WOMEN

GREG

WE COULDN'T GET OUT OF ANN ARBOR FAST ENOUGH. The good news was that my radiation and chemotherapy treatments were finally over; the bad news was that the doctors at the Cancer Center had nothing more to offer. I was told to follow up with a doctor in Traverse City and get another MRI taken of my head and neck in six months.

Ironically, I had felt so much better before going to the Cancer Center. Now I was in ghastly shape. The side effects of the chemo and radiation were devastating. I couldn't eat, I had lost a dangerous amount of weight, and I was in such extreme pain that I needed to take narcotics around the clock.

The side effects of the radiation continued. Just as sunburn doesn't stop cooking your skin the moment you cover yourself up and leave the beach, the burning of the tissue in my sinuses and mouth continued long after the rays stopped bombarding me. Even in the highly unlikely event that I survived, the radiation treatments themselves were carcinogenic and liable to cause yet another cancer in the future. That's because the rays might alter the DNA blueprint that was encoded in each of my cells, causing them to divide uncontrollably. After receiving such a whopping load of radiation during treatment, I was told I could never get another dose in my lifetime.

Even though the treatment almost killed me, I never questioned whether it was "worth it" or not. You might ask why anyone in their right mind would voluntarily walk through the gates of hell when even the cancer doctors admitted there was no known treatment. Our decision to go ahead with a toxic, destructive treatment with zero proven effectiveness was certainly against all odds. My experience at the Cancer Center was nightmarish, yet I still believed that Katherine and I made the right decision to do anything and everything we could to stop the tumor.

I refused to think about the future side effects of the radiation; I had my hands full worrying about the cancer. Most frightening to me was the prospect of the tumor destroying my brain. Would my memory be the first to go? Would the cancer eat away at my brain stem and paralyze me? What if I completely lost my mind?

My mind—what was left of it, anyway—returned to the days when I worked on a psychiatric unit. It was upsetting to see anyone suffer, but it was the folks who were truly out of their mind—the schizophrenics, manic-depressives, and the flipped-out patients on LSD—who really scared me. It was incredibly sad and disturbing to see them suffer, yet in all honesty I held a selfish comfort knowing that it was their problem. Now it was mine; I was the patient sick beyond repair, and there wasn't a damn thing I could do about it.

We drove through the grimy, crime-infested city of Flint as we made our way back home. In many respects, Flint seemed like a mirror image of me: once proud, bursting with life, the poster child for productivity and promise. Now Flint and I were rapidly decaying shells of our former selves. The wheels in my mind spun in unison with *Flow's* tires. Flint felt dead and gone, and I felt like I was heading in the same direction.

KATHERINE AND I AGREED that we would have a Fourth of July "celebration" at our lake home to mark the end of my treatment. The idea of having a party caught her between a rock and a hard place. On one hand she didn't think it would be good for me because I was worn out and in constant pain. On the other hand she somehow knew I needed a distraction. Finishing the treatment was a huge milestone for us, and we wanted to mark the occasion with friends who had helped us make it to the finish line. What we didn't discuss was the elephant in the room—that this Fourth of July was likely to be my last.

KATHERINE

THE FOURTH CAME WITH ALL ITS FANFARE. The crowds with their flag waving, noise making, and parades left me cold despite the heat of early July. It had never been my favorite holiday: it was extraneous at its best, idiotic at its worst. But this year was different; Greg's independence from the Cancer Center was worthy of commemorating. Our friends arrived throughout the day with their bowls of potato salad, homemade blueberry pie, coolers of cold drinks, and brown paper bags filled with hot dog buns, hamburgers, and all the fixings.

The most notable arrival was Jim and his son, Ben, who came with their car trunk filled with fireworks. They scurried about the yard, carefully lining up the explosives in the grass and building launching stations out of discarded lumber. I was afraid it would be too much for both Greg and me, but I put on my game face and ignored the anxious pit in my stomach. In reality, it didn't matter what I felt. This was Greg's celebration and there was no stopping him.

GREG

JIM AND HIS FAMILY CAME TO THE CELEBRATION in two cars that day, as his still newish *Highlander* was stuffed to the brim with the banned fireworks. My plate-throwing partners Kate and Mike drove up from Okemos to join us. Brenin and Emerson were happy to be back home with family friends. The Silver Lake cottage and Ann Arbor had become synonymous with cancer, hospitals, and dying, and we were all so happy to be 231 miles away from them.

Mike, Jim and I retreated to the basement workbench and attached several two-foot red tubes to a piece of scrap lumber. We carried the jerrybuilt contraption down to the lake and nailed it carefully to the end of the dock at a slight angle. This would insure that the shells would launch over the lake and not towards the house and spectators.

I watched as my family and our guests consumed the quintessential All-American Fourth of July barbecue. No one gave a big speech about why we were there that night; no one needed to. Although I was still in too much pain to swallow anything but the amber colored, narcotic-flavored shakes, I enjoyed being with my friends and family as they ate. I didn't envy them or feel self-pity as I watched them chow down the grilled hamburgers, hotdogs, and chips; I was just so grateful to be alive and to be with the people I loved.

KATHERINE

I STEPPED OUT INTO THE LONG RAYS of the afternoon sun with our friend Steve. He pushed back his cap and looked into the palms of his calloused hand. He reflected on all the months of chemo and radiation Greg had endured. "Their job was to push him right up to the edge, but not over it. Let's pray they got it right." His words, poignant and accurate, spoke to the fear I quietly carried. I could only stare up at him and nod my head.

We gathered around the overflowing picnic table, filled our plates, and bantered about the weather and summer plans. Then without direction, the crowd suddenly became silent. We knew beneath the frivolity why we were there. Over the months we had each carried a piece of Greg's battle, and the preciousness and precariousness of life had touched us all.

Now we stood together in Greg's presence. Our eyes registered for a moment his emaciated body and wisps of hair. We could feel his resilient, defiant sprit. It all came washing over us and we each stood a little taller to meet that spirit. Several of us found the words to express the love and the respect that we carried for him. We spoke simple gratitude for life itself, the lushness of summer, the breath in our lungs, and the support of one another. And then the feast began.

Everyone noticed, but no one commented, when Greg inconspicuously slipped into the bathroom to force down a small portion of the infamous shake. He knew his struggle to eat was almost as painful for his loved ones to watch as it was for him to swallow. When dusk turned to night and the fire pit glowed with embers, the show began.

GREG

SUDDENLY THE SHARP, CRACKING SOUND of firecrackers came from across the lake. Everyone took their positions on the deck, patio, and on old comforters strewn on the lakeside lawn. We took turns lighting the long green fuses on the shells and dropping them into the launching tubes. Once the fuses were lit, we ran towards the shore for safety and shouted, "Look out! Here she comes!" Sure enough, seconds later, the fuse would cough, sputter, and appear to die out. After a pause of a second or two, a loud thud would come from deep within the launcher, and, boy oh boy Houston, did we ever have ignition! The fiery shells rocketed up, screaming across the darkened sky like red shooting stars, and exploding into a bazillion brilliantly colored pieces that fell in an umbrella pattern into the lake. Each exploding shell was met by wild applause and yelling from the spectators.

Tears ran down my cheeks as the bursting fireworks lit up the night sky. Even though I was sick as a dog, it was one of the best days of my life. There I was, a little boy again in a grown-up body, surrounded by the love of my chosen family, celebrating my life with real fireworks. The best part about it was that the cancer woke me up from a lifelong slumber. No longer would I take anything—a hamburger, friends, fireworks, anything—for granted. That night I was more alive than ever before.

I felt like Cinderella. For a few hours I was transported from my miserable existence to a magical party filled with life and love. However, the clock struck twelve and our friends left one by one in their horsepower-driven carriages. The warm, enchanted evening dissolved, replaced immediately by the ice-cold reality of our suffering.

KATHERINE

WE WEREN'T PREPARED FOR WHAT CAME NEXT.

Greg did not feel his life returning. Instead, he felt weaker and sicker as each day passed. The radiation had created a destructive path within his cells. Like ninja warriors, the rays had slipped inside and stolen the integrity from both the cancerous and healthy cells. His exhaustion deepened, and he struggled to stay awake. His battle to eat was far from over, and he continued to fill a syringe with lidocaine and force down the liquid concoctions I created. Even sleep brought no respite. His breathing was raspy and labored. His throat and mouth were raw with pain, and bouts of night sweats drenched his T-shirt and sheets. The assault was unrelenting.

Our expectations, and those of our family, friends, and patients only made it worse. The treatment was over, right? Shouldn't he be getting better? We'd been warned in those first weeks that the side effects could worsen even after the treatments ended, but we had deliberately forgotten. Greg longed to return to some normalcy and mentioned returning to work. I was incredulous, and put my foot down; he could not work until he could eat.

All of this fueled my research for natural substances to assist in Greg's recovery. One plant I chanced upon was sea buckthorn. I had never heard of it before, but it has been used for thousands of years in Chinese medicine and had just recently been discovered by Western medicine. Clinical trials conducted throughout the last few decades confirmed the benefits ascribed to sea buckthorn oil in folk medicine.

As its name suggests, the plant thrives near coastlines, but it also grows in mountainous areas throughout the world. The medicinal properties are found in the oils of its red and golden berries. It heals skin damaged from UV exposure, burns, and radiation because of its high content of Vitamin A and E and their ability to squelch free radicals. Sea buckthorn reduces inflammation, helps cellular rejuvenation, and naturally boosts energy. Russian astronauts have used sea buckthorn oil to prevent UV rays from damaging their skin, while the Chinese use it in their burn and radiation clinics. If it was good enough for astronauts, it was good enough for Greg! I gave some of it to him in capsules, and applied a topical oil mixture directly to his neck and face.

It seemed to help! Two weeks into July, Greg began to rise like a phoenix from the ashes. He and Steve motored out on Lake Michigan, and Greg was reminded of his love for the water and his dreams of taking journeys through the Chain of Lakes. He relished the idea of being out in the open air and water with charts and maps, contemplating endless adventures. He excitedly confessed he wanted to go in with Steve on the purchase of the boat. I was totally surprised by the impulsivity of his plan. This was not the Greg I knew, but who was I to dictate the dreams of a sick man?

GREG

I KNEW I HAD TO FIND SOMETHING TO DO other than sit around the house feeling scared and depressed. Katherine needed to devote her time and energy toward building the medical practice of her dreams. She needed to spend less time worrying about me.

I reached out to my friend, Steve, a hardworking cherry farmer who helped take care of our lawn while we were in Ann Arbor. He was a tall, solidly built gentleman with thoughtful eyes and the manner to match. Steve had a strong mind and heart, a deep respect and connection to the land, and a quiet pride in managing his own affairs. Our relationship began obliquely through mutual friends, but as we got to know each other through golfing, beach barbecues, and watching college sports, we established a friendship of our own. We had gone through some of the rough patches of life together; I was there for him when his wife left, and now he was here for me when my world was unraveling.

Prior to my cancer diagnosis, we dreamed about purchasing a gently used boat and, when I was in Ann Arbor, Steve went ahead and made our dream a reality. He was eager to take me out for a spin. The *Laura Lynn* was a 24-foot beauty, big enough to handle the moderate seas of Lake Michigan, with an intimate cuddy cabin that could bunk down two people. Steve beamed as he helped me climb aboard, and proceeded to show me all the doodads. We fired up the big 350 horsepower V-8 engine and nosed the boat out of the harbor and into the bay. Steve hammered the throttle and we cut through the gentle waves on the lake like a knife through butter.

There's an axiom about boaters: the two best days of their lives are the day they purchase their boat and the day they sell it. It was great fun that day to be with my friend again and go bopping around the beautiful bay on our new used boat. Yet the more I thought about it, the more it became clear that I had just made one huge impulsive mistake. Steve was a big strong man with big strong trucks that could easily trailer the boat. I was a little weak guy, getting littler and weaker by the minute, with a faithful Subaru wagon that had all the heart, but none of the muscle to pull a boat.

I was bummed; the big fun on the big lake that I had imagined morphed into one big headache. It was hard to call Steve and tell him how I felt, but the truth of the matter was that another, better looking partner had come into his life, and her name was Sarah. They were gracious about buying out my share of the partnership, and the day that it happened was indeed one of my two best days owning the *Laura Lynn*.

That disappointing experience failed to cure my obsession with buying a boat, however. After all, if you live in northern Michigan on a lake, it follows that you have to own a boat. We had already owned a small, thirteen-foot Boston Whaler with hard wooden seats that gave our rear ends a good spanking every time we took it out. I wanted a more comfortable boat that we could sit in at the end of our dock, and, yes, I wanted one even though I didn't think I would live much longer. It was one of the few dreams that cancer had not taken away. I knew if I gave up all of my dreams I would be a goner for sure.

I made it a point to walk the two-mile loop that encircled our green-canopied peninsula each day. The combination of the cancer and the treatments whittled down my activity to three: lying down, sitting, or shuffling along the loop at a tortoise-like pace.

On one of my loops, I noticed a trailer with a boat on it covered with a brown canvas. There was a "FOR SALE" sign with a local phone number. I untied the cords that secured the canvas and discovered the object of my desire. Silver writing on the hull of the boat said it was a Sea Ray. She was all of 17 feet long, had real seats—the soft ones with fancy blue-and-white striped cushions—and her 135 horsepower V-6 engine had about a third of the gusto that *Laura Lynn* had. Yet that was all the gusto I needed. I called the owner and bought the boat a few days later. It was one of my two happiest days owning the Sea Ray.

Katherine offered no objection to all my scurrying about buying and selling boats. She seemed happy I was doing something other than sitting around and worrying about the cancer. We had talked previously about my life and whether there was anything "left" that I wanted to do. It was a subtle shift, acknowledging that we were nearing the end. We never went as far as calling it my "bucket list" as that would have meant waving the white towel. Katherine wasn't surprised to hear that I didn't want to take any special trips, or do something nutty like parachute out of an airplane. In all honesty, I couldn't imagine taking any trip; I had my hands full simply ambling around our peninsula.

KATHERINE

THERE WERE MOMENTS WHEN I GREW WEARY of his illness dominating every waking moment and interrupting my sleep. I struggled to find a corner of solitude where I could focus on my own life and glimpse some kind of future. Yet his symptoms continued without end. As soon as one resolved, a new one appeared and became equally distressing. It frustrated me that there was rarely even an acknowledgement that the old one had gotten better now that the new one demanded our attention.

I began to understand the expression "the patience of Job," and was impressed by the man's incredible faith. During his lifetime he experienced unbelievable loss as his animals—thousands of them— were destroyed and his children killed. He was then besieged by his own illness, with boils and sores covering his entire body. Talk about being "tested"! Even then he did not curse his life or his God. Perhaps I was emulating Job when I would tell myself, "Just be with what is happening. Embrace it more fully. Savor even this."

Yet on many days, I didn't understand why Greg and I were being tested. I dug deep to find a reservoir of faith. Would I be deterred by the magnitude of his problems? Would I become overwhelmed by the seriousness? This was our fate and our experience to live. I refused to feel vindictive.

I remembered the day when we'd thrown dishes against the garage wall. For some reason, I couldn't connect with my anger that day. But the idea still sounded good, and I tried a plate or two. It brought me no relief. The truth was that sometimes I did feel angry, but more than anger I felt fear. And more than the fear, I felt challenged and compelled to grow, to fight, and to evolve. I took the path of Job and contemplated the words of Robert Frost, "The best way out is always through."

GREG

I APPROACHED THE PLATE OF FOOD WITH CAUTION. The pain in my mouth was less intense and I gathered my courage to try a bite. I ate the eggs in the only way I could that evening—in tiny bites and in slow motion. The cancer and treatment side effects now demanded that I make heightened awareness, or mindfulness, my number one priority. The eggs and the two strawberries that accompanied them slid down the hatch, and it didn't hurt! We both began to cry.

Several years back, we went on two retreats with the Vietnamese monk Thich Nhat Hanh and studied the art of mindful living. He talked about the importance of slowing down, the miracle of living in the present moment and gradually increasing our awareness of each and every step. One exercise during the retreat was to eat an apple, savoring each individual bite. Katherine and I were impressed with his teachings; like most Americans we had been speeding down the stressed-out fast track.

Slowing down and being fully present was not my long suit. It was impossible for me to get the hang of meditation as my mind used it as an opportunity to be anywhere but in the here and now. After many failed attempts I came up with a solution: I would stop trying to tell my mind what other people thought it should do, and just let it go wherever it wanted during meditation. It was so relaxing to sit on the dark blue cushion and free my mind of restrictions, no matter where they came from.

As I carefully chewed the eggs that night, the thought crossed my mind for the first time that someday I might be able to eat again. My eyes welled with tears at the thought, and then my mind bolted from the table and raced away into the distant future: if I could start eating, then I might be able to…It wasn't nearly the end of the shakes that day, but I began to see faint glimpses of an imagined future through my watery eyes.

KATHERINE

THE CLEARING SKIES AND THE MOIST EARTH beckoned us outside. The spirea was a vibrant pink and in full bloom amidst the fragrant lavender. It was almost too much for me to bear. Almost. Greg and I strolled through the yard and onward around the two-mile loop through the neighborhood. Walking hand in hand, we teased each other and swung our arms like young lovers. I noticed Greg's slow steps and baggy clothes, but my heart defied my eyes. It could see what my eyes could not. I whispered to myself, "Heaven is now, heaven is here."

Later that night Greg took an Epsom salt bath and I rubbed his neck and feet with lotion despite great fuss and protest. The joy of the afternoon walk faded and was replaced by his worries. His ear felt "full" on the left side and there was growing pressure from nasal congestion. Fear was scratching at the door again—fear of the tumor growing, returning, and destroying him. We went to bed and slept a few hours only to be awakened by his cries for help. I turned on the light and found him drenched in sweat and gasping for air. We changed his T-shirt and pillowcase, and I put my arm gently around him until he slipped back into sleep.

What did it all mean? I lay there awake in the empty hours of night and my sadness found me again. Undefended, I considered the possibility that there would be no turning back from Greg's steady decline, his disability, and his death. I shivered as this dark thought settled into me. Yet right beside that possible outcome, there emerged one that promised recovery. It carried the miracle of spirit, of life, of intentional healing. I knew there would be love either way.

I reaffirmed my commitment to help Greg live. We agreed to continue to do everything that we had begun: the medicinal mushrooms, the probiotics, the whey protein, the vitamins and minerals, the essential fatty acids, and the proteolytic enzymes three times a day with all the plant antioxidants, including the curcumin, grape-seed extract, green tea extract, boswelian, and milk thistle.

We were not going to back down. The standard cancer treatments bombarded the cancer, but they did nothing to nurture or restore life. I turned to Eastern medicine, and believed that acupuncture and herbs could help replenish his depleted energy, his chi, and his yin deficiency. In the darkness that surrounded us, I vowed silently to share whatever I had learned with others, be they patients, friends, or strangers.

After eating his first solid meal, Greg began to return to work for a few hours each day. We acted out the charade of normalcy. It wasn't exactly lying. We were eager to put the cancer behind us, and so we fumbled about like beginners on the dance floor. Unsure of our steps, we faked it, trying to pretend that things were heading back to normal.

GREG

EVEN THOUGH KATHERINE HAD MADE AN EXHAUSTIVE effort to find the right combination of therapies, I had an intuition that we both needed something more.

My epiphany came while I was ruminating on the Chinese symbol for yin and yang, a deceptively simple looking circle consisting of a white and black tear drop shape with contrasting dots. The black teardrop is a symbol for yin, or feminine energy, whereas the white teardrop represents yang, or masculine energy. I remembered in Jungian psychology, as well as from a flirting acquaintance with Taoist philosophy, how "ultimate power," or harmony, came only when those two life forces were in balance with one another. I've witnessed the power of this philosophy at work in many of my patients. People would often continue to be distressed until they became familiar, or "got in touch," with the unexpressed side of themselves.

I knew my cancer treatment was way out of whack. It wasn't that the approach the cancer doctors used was bad, we just needed something to complement—or balance—what I saw as an overly masculine approach, one that left no room for tenderness or emotion. Katherine exuded this complementary energy, but she couldn't do it alone. She needed the support and nurturance from others as much as I did.

An image from our trip to New Zealand returned to help me.

One day we took a daylong excursion from our cottage in Hahei, a small village nestled along the seashore of the North Island. We drove inland through the Kauri forest and felt inspired by the ancient trees. We traveled on to Waterworks Park, a quirky spot set among five acres of beautiful Coromandel bush, far from the hustle and bustle of any town. The place was filled with water-powered toys. Bicycles squirted water out of their handlebars as you peddled them, and a wooden water clock kept amazingly accurate time.

We were meandering down a shady dirt path with Emerson in her stroller, heading for the zip-line, when I happened to look deeper into the bush. I spied something peculiar that was partially hidden in the thick undercover. Curious, I walked to the side of the trail, parted the bushes, and was startled to discover several bronze, life-size statues of women sitting in a circle. The women strongly resonated with something deep inside me, and I beckoned Katherine and Emerson to come over and look at what I had found.

KATHERINE

I LOOKED CLOSELY THROUGH THE CAMOUFLAGE of the shaded forest. The women were seated in a circle, cross-legged and meditating, their hands folded in their laps. They were similar in posture, but with subtle differences in their dress and hair. Their simplicity in the undisturbed silence was riveting. In the center of their circle was a plate-sized, white quartz stone which starkly contrasted with the women's brown bodies. The image held my gaze, but Greg was totally captivated.

Months later, after he completed his chemotherapy and radiation, Greg confided to me, "I want to have a healing ceremony of women. Remember the sculpture we saw in New Zealand? Like that. A circle of women healers we know." I agreed to help make it happen. And as mid-July crested, I planned the ceremony.

GREG

I FINALLY UNDERSTOOD WHY the circle of the women statues had touched me that day in New Zealand. I now needed their power, strength, and grace.

Katherine was all for the idea, and six women from various walks of life accepted our invitation. We gathered on a perfect July afternoon. At first, the women sat in silence on the red Oriental rug in our living room. I lay face up in the middle of the group, a pillow under my head.

The rule that day was that there were no rules. Honestly, I can't remember much of what followed. I do remember the women sitting with a quiet dignity in a meditative circle, just like the bronze statues among the ferns of New Zealand. Each person took a turn offering meditations, leading chants, and saying prayers.

KATHERINE

THE TALKING STOPPED, and we placed our hands upon Greg's body. Sandy, a yoga therapist, took out her Tibetan singing bowl and brought forth its deep resonance by running the edge of the bowl with its striker. The vibration filled the space in our hearts, minds, and bodies. It resonated until there was no separation within or between us.

Without warning the sky darkened, and a loud crack of thunder broke through the silence. The wind picked up and a storm moved across the lake. Each woman held herself open to the intention of being a healing presence; each soul became an instrument for the highest good. Slowly we lifted Greg's body off the red rug and held him in the circle of our arms. Intelligence and energy flowed through us without doubt or hesitation.

Suddenly a dam broke within me as the lightening flashed. I realized the ceremony was for me, too, and tears streamed down my face. I released what I had carried alone for months—the fear, the exhaustion, and the desperation. As Greg's body rocked weightless in our arms, I yielded to the boundless support of the women and God. An immense weight lifted from my shoulders, and only as it left, did I realize its magnitude. Greg's body was gently lowered to the ground. We rested in quiet silence as the storm moved through the room and onward down the lake.

As if waking from a dream, Greg slowly sat up and looked sleepily upon us. We sat together in silence and refrained from small talk. We had transcended the realm of words and no one wanted to alter the sanctity that surrounded us.

GREG

I'D LIKE TO TELL YOU that after the ceremony was over I jumped up, yelled "Hallelujah!" and was completely cured. If only that were true! What actually happened was that I hugged all the women with a deep sense of gratitude. We said goodbye amidst tears and their assurances that I was going to "make it." A few women remarked that the thunder was a "good sign." Then they left.

What I remember the most was how everyone gave of herself so freely that day, and how I allowed myself to receive love unconditionally. But instead of feeling better after the ceremony, I took a turn that night for the worse. The sinus area on the left side of my face was throbbing and congested, and I was scared about the increased inflammation. It was difficult to breathe and my left ear began to ache.

I took my nightly Klonopin chill pill in an effort to put out the forest fire of anxiety that was raging through my mind, I couldn't remember the last time I had actually had a good night's sleep. Worry is a terrible bed partner, and terror is the very worst. My recurring dream of being in an airplane crash spooked me once again that night:

I'm flying on a huge jet, and I have a feeling that something is wrong. I look out the small, oval window and see that the plane is flying dangerously low over the hilly streets of San Francisco. I'm filled with dread as the plane goes into a nose-dive towards a street. But the jet miraculously comes to a landing. I jump off the airplane and frantically run around, trying to find a phone. I am sure the plane crash was on CNN, and I want everyone to know I am okay.

I woke up drenched in sweat. Why did I always have stupid dreams about planes crashing? I tried to free associate to the different parts of the dream, just as I would instruct my psychotherapy patients to do. Jet? Flying? Up in the air? My mind raced as I tried to piece together the associations: a jet, in trouble, bridge, landing on a street, CNN, no phone, the need to let everyone know I'm okay? What a jumbled mess! No wonder I'd worked up such a sweat!

My face was still swollen that morning, and it was difficult for me to breathe. Katherine helped me change the damp sheets, and I went into the bathroom to look at my face. I rotated my head slowly to the left, then right, carefully scanning the reflection in the mirror to see if my left cheek looked puffier than the right. There were no obvious differences. Katherine tried to reassure both of us that the swelling was likely the result of the radiation treatment, rather than proof that the tumor was growing. I so much wanted to believe her.

I didn't need another MRI; what I needed was faith. I had complete confidence in Katherine and knew she was trying to do everything she could to help me. But I needed to believe we would find a way to defeat the cancer and that I would live!

20.

HOLY GRAILS

GREG

PEOPLE IN THE COMMUNITY continued to reach out and let us know they were thinking about us. Karen Gillhooly, a local rheumatologist, sent me a copy of the book *Long Life,* by Mary Oliver, with a beautiful bookmark made from amber glass beads. Karen was very involved with the local Montessori school, and she enjoyed my presentations to the school's staff at their annual retreats. I frequently included poems in the lectures, including Oliver's "Wild Geese," which became a staff favorite. Karen strategically placed the bookmark to mark Oliver's essay on Ralph Waldo Emerson. She knew that he was our daughter's namesake. There was no need for a card; the title of the book and the chapter said it all. I only hoped that I could have a long life with Emerson!

An intriguing piece of correspondence came from a stranger, Nancy, who wrote that she'd tried to contact Katherine several weeks ago when she first heard about my diagnosis. She recommended that I arrange an appointment with Libby Slocum, an acupuncturist and alternative healer with an office in Kalamazoo.

Nancy wrote in her follow-up letter that she was "not the kind of person who usually bothers people." She mentioned that Libby had saved her life, and believed that she could help me, too. She ended the letter on a somewhat cryptic note by writing: "You'll know why you're meeting with Libby the minute you meet her."

Katherine was reluctant to act on Nancy's unsolicited advice and arrange an appointment with Libby. I understood how she felt; a large part of me didn't want to leave the sanctuary of our home. After barely surviving weeks at the Cancer Center, not to mention asking Katherine and Brenin to put their lives on hold to take care of me, traveling downstate to meet with some stranger, perhaps a quack, was on par with a root canal.

Yet I had an intuition that we should go, and I presented my case to Katherine. At the end of the day the bottom-line was this: What did we have to lose? After all, no one else had any better idea of what we should do! What if this Nancy "knew" something? Katherine finally relented, and we packed up *Flow* and hit the road again, this time heading to my childhood home in Grand Rapids.

KATHERINE

FITTING IN A VISIT TO LIBBY SEEMED UNREALISTIC with the million and one details of life. But Greg wanted to try. Libby and I had spoken several months ago on the telephone, and I was struck then by the amount of time she spent sharing her helpful ideas. She radiated hope, which we desperately needed, so we scheduled an appointment to go to her office on Saturday.

The doctors at the University of Michigan had done all they could do. Their farewell instructions were simple: get examined by the local ENT physician and have a repeat PET scan in six months. Dr. Noorgard, the ENT who had examined Greg in March, was on medical leave and seriously ill with pancreatic cancer. Greg's internist was worried and sympathetic, but had nothing else to offer. So one month after treatment we were totally on our own. I desperately wanted someone to help guide us, or to at least review the program I had created over the months.

And so the path emerged. We stayed with Greg's parents who still lived independently in their family home in Grand Rapids. Greg's sister, Laura, and niece, Stephanie, were thrilled to babysit Emerson. We drove down Friday night for an early dinner and to help Emerson become acclimated once again to the extended Holmes clan.

GREG

THEY SAY YOU CAN NEVER GO HOME AGAIN; I say that's not true. In many ways we never leave home—we carry it squarely on our backs like turtles as we move through life. Our memories and feelings about home remain imprinted deep within us, no matter how far away we travel or what new "shell" we inhabit later in our lives.

When we arrived in the northeastern suburbs of Grand Rapids, I discovered that my childhood shell had remained virtually intact. There was a museum-like quality to the modest ranch home, everything preserved just as I remembered it 30-plus years ago when I left for college. All that was missing were red velvet ropes and a docent to recount the family history. There was the living room that my mother had burst into when she demanded that my friends and I leave the country because we disagreed with her politics. The rocking chair where my father sat while we watched the boxing matches remained in the living room. Some of the rooms had been gussied up a bit with a roll of wallpaper or a splash of paint, but not much else was different.

My parents were startled when I came through the garage door and entered the kitchen. They looked as though they were seeing a ghost, and I probably looked like one; I wasn't much more than a bag of bones. It frightened me to look at myself in a mirror, and I could only imagine what my parents felt.

I wasn't the only person in the room who had changed. My parents had aged considerably over the past few years, and it seemed to me that they were beginning their descent. My mother's chronic struggles with illness and medications had taken the starch out of her long ago, and now she was slowly losing command of her mind. She had called family members by the wrong names for years, and I'm sure it didn't help matters one bit when we imitated her miscues. My mother enjoyed making fun of our mistakes as much as anyone. She may not have taught us how to tease each other, but she did nothing to teach us to draw the line between affectionate teasing and humiliation. I must admit I felt a mixture of sadness, satisfaction, and guilt when I watched her get a dose of her own medicine.

My family stayed in character that afternoon. I didn't want to upset them, and it was clear that they didn't want to upset me. It was the way we were and the way we would always be. Katherine and I explained that we were going to see someone in Kalamazoo for a "consultation," without further discussion.

We said our goodbyes the next morning and headed down the interstate to meet Libby. Katherine basked in the early rays of light spilling through the car window. My thoughts were all over the place, and none of them were positive. For the first few miles I wondered what the heck I was doing. Why did I bug Katherine to go see Libby? Katherine embraced alternatives to traditional medicine, but I felt that she was skeptical about what Libby could offer. My guilt continued to snowball as I thought about all the hardships I was putting her through.

We pulled off the freeway and turned into a garden-variety office park located on the outer edge of Kalamazoo. The fact that there were no cars in the large parking lot added temporary fuel to the fire of my doubts until I remembered it was early Saturday morning. As we looked around the low-slung buildings to verify that we were in the right place, a car pulled up beside us.

KATHERINE

A PETITE WOMAN with short, sandy brown hair bounced out of the car. Dressed in sea-blue linen that matched her eyes, she strode quickly across the asphalt and extended her hand to welcome us. I knew immediately from her energetic handshake that we were in for an adventure.

We entered her office, where she switched the lights on, revealing an open-style waiting room with tasteful art on pastel walls. The morning light filtered through the windows, illuminating shelves of well-used books. Rocking chairs and weathered armchairs were in small clusters around the room. It spoke volumes about her style of practice. Here was a mixing pot for sharing stories, time, and ideas. The office couldn't have felt more different from the cold, minimalistic doctors' offices we had come to know.

I don't think my mouth was gaping, but I felt so relieved that my body language was surely saying, "Finally! Finally someone we can talk to without censorship and ridicule!" As we told our story, Libby seemed unruffled by the complexity and seriousness of Greg's illness. Small details and impressions were as important to her as the diagnosis and pathology report.

After our interview, Libby wanted to give Greg a traditional acupuncture treatment. We entered a room with an examination table, a few chairs, and a beautiful silk screen on the wall. He stretched out on the exam table, cushioned and warm with soft flannel sheets. Libby took his pulse and deftly inserted her needles. As she did so, she quietly explained to me the name of the point and the purpose for which she chose them: kidney 6, 27, and 3; lung 7; spleen 4; and local sinus points. Greg surrendered easily to her direction and teased us about his problems requiring two acupuncturists . I sensed that he trusted Libby immediately. With needles in place, he fell into a light sleep.

The acupuncture session proved to be only the tip of the iceberg of Libby's un-Westernized view of medicine and healing. At the end of the session, the three of us discussed other possible treatments. Acupuncture would continue to be a key part of our plan, along with supplements that she agreed to review.

Then Libby introduced us to the third part of the plan: a low-level laser light that she wheeled in on a silver metal tray. She explained the basic physics of lasers: How they emit polarized light, essentially photons of light which move in a coherent wave. This is in contrast to everyday light, which scatters in a myriad of directions and different wave formations. She mentioned the research that explained how lasers helped tissues heal. Individual cells are able to take up the coherent light in such a way that it energizes their mitochondria to create ATP. This important molecule, ATP, holds the phosphate bonds that store and release energy for the cell to use in a million different ways. My own reading supported that theory. The final enzyme in the production of ATP, technically known as cytochrome c oxidase, appears to accept energy from laser-level lights.

The research I had done suggested that doses of Low Level Laser Therapy (LLLT) reduced pain by lowering the influx of white blood cells and other molecules that created inflammation. This enabled the cells to heal by moving from injury and inflammation toward repair. The best clinical research involved placebo-controlled studies with people who developed overuse injuries from repetitive movements working on assembly lines. There was also research using the laser for carpel tunnel complaints in individuals with rheumatoid arthritis. It was cheaper than surgery and, for some people, quite effective.

We were open to trying the laser, and were relieved to know there were no hidden side effects. We also fully understood that there was no guarantee. At this point we had nothing to lose, and potentially so much to gain.

She then described the body in a new way. In Chinese medicine, the abdomen has specific areas corresponding to each acupuncture meridian. By directing the laser to these areas, you could influence the particular organ that lies beneath the skin—the spleen, the liver, the stomach—and also the meridians flowing throughout the body. I was fascinated. Libby held the laser diode directly on Greg's belly and moved it every three to five minutes. Greg lay there in a state of relaxed receptivity.

As we ended our first visit, she recommended we return the next day for a follow-up appointment, and asked if we could bring the bottles of supplements for her to review more carefully. We were grateful for her willingness to see us in a way that accommodated our schedules.

We were amazed that four hours had passed so quickly. We had found an ally and a resource in our new acquaintance. It was too early to confirm, but already Libby felt like a friend and a healer. I appreciated another set of eyes and ears to tend to Greg, and valued some, if not all, of her ideas. Most importantly, Greg seemed renewed from their interaction. Libby gave us a big hug and waved a fervent goodbye as I babied Flow out of the parking lot. On the ride back to Grand Rapids we talked about our morning. We agreed the visit was a greatly needed breath of fresh air. It couldn't have been more different from our appointments at the Cancer Center.

Emerson was ecstatic when we returned to Greg's parents' house. Stephanie had spent the morning introducing her to the Barbie doll collection from her not so distant childhood, along with numerous small suitcases filled with innumerable dress-up outfits. Emerson was eager to show me all her treasures. Greg settled in the family room, sinking into the sofa and attempting to field questions about how the morning had gone. The experience was something he couldn't easily explain, and thankfully his family didn't press for specifics. They were content that we were there, and happy to know he was doing his best to put some weight back on. Details were not their forte. Instead they focused on their favorite card games, and we cheerfully joined in.

GREG

OUR APPOINTMENT SUNDAY MORNING turned out to be as strange and interesting as Saturday's. We met Libby once again in the empty parking lot, where she greeted us with a carton of chicken eggs. "Here," she said, with more than a hint of pride in her voice. "This is a present from my girls." I assumed her daughters had collected the eggs from a chicken coop, but it turned out that her "girls" were the hens that laid the eggs.

Libby gave me another acupuncture treatment that morning, during which I fell asleep. After the treatment was finished, Libby pricked our fingers with a tiny needle and took samples to determine our respective blood types. She firmly believed in the controversial theory that people with different blood types require different types of nutrition. I had an O blood type, and she inquired as to the kind of foods we ate. When Katherine and I told her that we were on a low-fat, vegetarian diet, Libby appeared alarmed and stated flat out that the diet was hurting me.

I was startled by Libby's conclusion. Katherine and I had spent an enormous amount of time and energy following a "healthy" diet, one devoid of all the evil fats that doctors claimed were the culprits of heart disease. Newly converted, we had gone on to preach the gospel to our patients over the next several years. How could a "healthy" diet be bad for you, and vice versa? Libby explained that whereas our "grain-based" diet was perfect for Katherine, an A blood type, O blood types require a different diet. She suggested that I change my diet immediately, and eat the foods that my body was "calling for."

Libby offered a few examples of foods she believed were "call-ing" me: beef, snapper, olive oil, walnuts, garlic, onions, mangos, and blueberries. In retrospect, none of these foods, except for the beef, contained "evil" oils, and I was eating most of them anyway—at least I had been before my cancer. What amazed me was that I craved every one of the foods and spices that she mentioned. A couple of them could even provoke a Pavlovian-like salivary response. Libby was convinced that we crave certain foods because our body "knows" we need them. Katherine could care less about eating a steak, for example, whereas the smell of a juicy Delmonico sizzling on a neighbors' grill could bring me to tears.

To "test" which supplements might be beneficial for me, Libby asked me to hold a bottle in a fist close to my body, and try to resist her attempts to pull my arm forward. She referred to this litmus test as "muscle testing."

It sounded bizarre, and I must admit it was difficult to suspend my skepticism. How could my muscles "know" what supplements I needed to take? I was familiar with the concept of muscle memo-ry, phenomena that occurs when movement is repeated over time and can be performed without conscious effort, such as riding a bike, typing on a keyboard, and playing video games. But believing that muscles "know" what vitamins you need was difficult to swal-low. However, at that point I was willing to try just about anything, so I grabbed the small white bottles one by one, flexed what little muscles remained in my right arm, moved it toward my chest, and attempted to resist Libby's best efforts to pull my arm forward.

I couldn't believe what happened next. When I held some of the bottles in my hand, I could easily resist Libby's efforts to pull my arm back, when I held others, my muscles surrendered.

Libby agreed with most of the supplements I was taking, but wanted to add one that addressed yin deficiency. From Katherine's study of acupuncture, I knew of the importance of balancing the yin and the yang forces—a sophisticated yet elemental concept which forms the basic foundation of Eastern thought. The yin force provides nurturance—the cooling, moistening, restorative force—while the yang offers the warming, energizing, active dimension. Yin deficiency was thought to contribute to many chronic diseases, especially cancer. Traditional cancer therapies are very yang and further aggravate any underlying yin deficiency. Libby prescribed a mixture of herbs to strengthen yin, which would aid my sleep, decrease my night sweats, and increase the absorption of nutrients from food.

Despite my good feelings toward Libby, I wondered whether I was just another desperate cancer victim ready to part with my money for false hope. An herbal supplement to nourish my yin deficiency? That crazy thing with glass bottles and energy? And what about the controversy of blood type and diet? I thought about my brothers and sisters in arms, hundreds of thousands of young and old people tormented by cancers of their own, forced to go on their respective death marches. Most of them were people just like me—good souls, really—people with no option other than the conventional treatment.

Cancer, with its looming specter of a long and painful death, often creates an unusual mixture of vulnerability and resolve that is difficult to describe. I used to wonder what people like the actor Steve McQueen were thinking when they ran off to Mexico to get Laetrile treatments for their cancer. Like most people, I thought he was just another victim of "voodoo medicine." But that was before I had a cancer of my own. I now saw his eleventh-hour pursuit in a totally different light. The only difference between the two of us was that he went off to Mexico to pursue the Holy Grail, while I downed Katherine's shakes and supplements and went off to Kalamazoo.

Libby's pitch to me about blood types and diet was compelling, even though I was aware that it was highly controversial. When Libby first mentioned the diet, I remembered the heart problems that came to light shortly after switching to an extremely low fat diet. It began in the middle of one night when a sharp, momentary pain in my chest woke me up. I screamed out to Katherine for help as I clutched my chest. The intense pain scared the crap out of both of us, although it stopped as suddenly as it began. I begged Katherine to take my pulse and she attempted to assure me (unsuccessfully) that I was not having a heart attack, even though my pulse was irregular.

After several weeks of these periodic "attacks," a cardiologist suggested I wear a 24-hour halter monitor to see if it could capture my nighttime symptoms. Katherine and the cardiologist reviewed the results from the EKG and concluded that something was happening to me in the middle of the night, but at the end of the day all the cardiologist could honestly say was that it was not life threatening. He sent me for a stress test to determine if there was underlying heart disease. The test was "negative," and the cardiologist concluded that I had frequent premature ventricular contractions (PVC), a "benign" condition.

There was one problem. When I did "throw a PVC" now and then, it was painless. His diagnosis failed to explain the excruciating episodes that I suffered in the middle of the night. It wasn't all that significant—to him, anyway. The periodic attacks never did stop. Every time the sharp pain woke me, I would grab at my left ribcage and try to tell myself that there was nothing to worry about. I wasn't convincing.

Finally, in a panic, I'd wake up Katherine, who would take my pulse and tell me that I was NOT having a heart attack. Time and time again she came to my nocturnal rescue without complaint. I had serious doubts about my heart, but I had absolutely none about hers.

KATHERINE

I THOUGHT ABOUT LIBBY'S ENDORSEMENT of a diet based on blood type, and paused. My own dietary blueprint was designed from a unique mixture of theories. I had been a proponent of a plant-based diet since high school when I read, *Diet for a Small Planet* by Francis Moore Lappe. It is important to me that everyone eat in a way that supports the whole planet, and without consuming vast resources in the production of food. A diet based on meat was possible only through clear cutting forests and draining aquifers to grow the grain to feed the cattle. I strongly believed we needed to get our diets off the top of the food chain.

In truth, I had grown up a little "protein phobic," like many young vegetarians. Over the years I learned healthy ways to consume quality protein, and wasn't completely opposed to eating meat, but I knew it was a slippery slope. Too much protein, such as the Atkins diet, was just plain bad for the dieter and the environment. Bring on the burger, but hold the bun and slather on the cheese and bacon. Yikes. But what about diet for cancer?

I was particularly interested in the recommendations of Nicholas Gonzales, M.D. In Gonzales' opinion, patients with solid epithelial tumors—such as tumors of the lung, pancreas, colon, prostate, uterus, etc.—do best on a largely plant-based diet. Such patients have a metabolism that functions most efficiently with a specific combination of nutrients that are found in fruits, vegetables, nuts, whole grains and seeds, and minimal to no animal protein. Allowed are daily eggs and fish protein once or twice per week.

On the other hand, he believed patients with blood or immune-based malignancies such as leukemia, myeloma and lymphoma do best on a high-animal protein, high-fat diet. He recommended that their diets be based on animal products, with minimal to moderate amounts of plant-based foods.

His recommendations stemmed from how diet affects the patient's nervous system. A plant-based diet is found to support the calming parasympathetic nervous system and the animal-based diet strengthens the sympathetic. Because Greg had a solid tumor in the sinus area, the ideal diet for him was plant-based, with some allowable proteins.

Equally important, his diet should contain good oils from fish, nuts, avocados, and limited refined carbohydrates. One of the best ways to limit inflammation is by getting the sugar and saturated, hydrogenated fats out of the diet. Eliminating white flour and sugar was a household goal. Greg embraced the sugar restriction with enthusiasm, much to Emerson's sweet-toothed (and mine to a smaller degree) chagrin. We sought an organic, plant-based diet that offered quality protein and few, if any, pesticides. I fine-tuned our selection of grains, vegetables, and proteins by studying the foods that supported a yin deficiency.

As Libby tested Greg by holding each bottle to his chest and then pushing against his resisting outstretched arm, I remembered how I had poured over books and scoured the Internet for the information that led me to these supplemental recommendations. Could it really be this easy? I had seen other people test supplements this way, and had even experienced it personally over the years. I had tried, out of curiosity, to perform such muscle tests on family and friends but always felt disappointed. I could never get a clear reproducible response that I could be confident in, so I didn't pursue it further. Just because I couldn't feel things that other people were capable of feeling, I didn't outright dismiss it. I attended several courses at MSU College of Osteopathic Medicine and was always amazed at the palpatory skills of their discipline. They could detect the subtle muscle tension patterns and positions of ribs and vertebrae that escaped me.

So as I watched Libby, I trusted that she knew what she felt and what it meant to her. Although I valued her input, I knew I wouldn't stop the nutrients that I had selected and believed were right for Greg's condition.

Good medicine is often intuitive. I wasn't wholly confident, for example, about things I was trying at the recommendation of an herbalist, including the use of pawpaw, a common plant used in cancer from a tree native to the Midwest. I knew it could affect energy production in both cancer cells as well as healthy cells, making it a doubled-edged sword. Was this a net gain or net loss? My intuition was that it wasn't helping Greg, and this feeling was reinforced by Libby's muscle testing. But would I stop curcumin based on her tests? No way! My research on this was substantial and solid. I appreciated what Libby could sense in the same way I trusted osteopaths and energy healers. There was room in my paradigm for energy, subjectivity, and intuition. But in the end, I had to trust my own wisdom. I thought back to a comment I'd made during an interview as a medical school applicant: *Modern medicine does not have a monopoly on healing.*

LOW LEVEL LASER THERAPY LINKS

- http://www.ncbi.nlm.nih.gov/pubmed/22450151
- http://www.ncbi.nlm.nih.gov/pubmed/12775206
- http://www.spectramedics.com/index.php?id=101
- http://en.wikipedia.org/wiki/Low_level_laser_therapy

As the visit was wrapping up, I hesitantly mentioned that my right shoulder felt tight, and explained that I might have lifted a suitcase incorrectly. She put one hand on my tense muscles and said, "Your turn!" Soon I was on the table and experiencing a technique known as Qua Sha. She gently rubbed my back with Tiger Balm. Its aroma soon filled the room and my sinuses with pungent clove and menthol. She scraped the ointment off my clenched muscles with the edge of a Chinese soupspoon. Ouch! It certainly wasn't relaxing, at least not at first. I fought the urge to yell or burst out laughing—the sensation was that intense. So I clenched my teeth in a grimace and felt my muscles gradually soften and release. So this was what it took for me to settle down! I laughed for days when I remembered the strange mixture of pleasure and pain. Would I always need to be arm wrestled into relaxing?

SEVERAL WEEKS AFTER SEEING LIBBY, I made the decision to purchase a laser, and registered for a course in Chicago to further explore its science and application. Now I would be able to provide my own version of treatment to Greg several times a week in the comfort of our home. We managed to work it into our weekly schedule, and gradually created an odd family ritual.

I would look at Greg at the end of a busy day and see the exhaustion hanging over him like a cloud. I felt his body and spirit calling out for help to stop the downward spiral. I would casually say, "How about a treatment?" and coax him down the stairs of our split-level home.

Soon he was stretched out on the floor with cushions and bolsters, and I would place a steaming hot washcloth over his eyes and sinus area. The moist heat sent a wave of relaxation over him, and encouraged the blood to flow to his face and nose. After taking his pulse, I would create the best acupuncture needle combination I could imagine for him at that moment. I pushed through my insecurity and listened with my heart. Greg needed to receive and I needed to give; we surrendered to the call for healing.

Once the needles were in place, I began the laser treatment with special attention directed to his internal organs. I sat beside him on the floor and passed the laser over his belly. It made a little beep with each joule of energy it emitted. There were no words between us or within me. It was a time of mindfulness, of prayer, and of love.

As I worked, Emerson sat above us on the futon and wiggled her toes against my neck. She liked watching a particular segment of the *Wizard of Oz* with the volume turned down, but she would often jump down and join us on the floor to make sure everything was all right. Invariably, Greg would fall asleep and begin to snore deeply. Emerson and I would smile and giggle at the sounds her daddy could make.

21.

LIVING IN PARADISE

GREG

I WOULD GRIT MY TEETH whenever I thought about Katherine's struggle to be taken seriously. She tried so hard to win the acceptance of her colleagues and was constantly rebuffed. Katherine was a throwback to a different era of medicine when Marcus Welby-type doctors made house calls, unhurriedly inquiring about your family, pets, and garden, while treating you with respect.

I felt horrible that our battle with cancer demanded most of Katherine's time and attention. This was supposed to be her time to lay claim to something for herself. I wanted so badly for her to have her own practice. She had fought long and hard to be herself in a medical world that rejected her. Now her dreams were put on hold as she was trying to save me.

We talked frequently about her frustrations, and her dreams, and I encouraged her not to stop pursuing them just because I had cancer. I reminded her of the grim reality that if I died she would still need to work. Why not practice in a place she really wanted to be? I only wished that I could live long enough to see it.

I HAD MIXED FEELINGS ABOUT RETURNING to my own practice. I'd been off work for a few months, and a part of me was eager to start again. I missed my patients, and I knew from their cards and letters that they missed me. I offered to refer my orphaned clients to other psychologists, yet none took me up on it.

Was it fair to my patients if I went back to work? They deserved the spotlight, not me! How would they feel about their problems when they compared them to mine? My cancer was already ruining several lives, and I didn't want its tentacles to spread to my patients. On the other hand, was it right for me to try to control their actions? Would I be taking away an important opportunity for them to see me and to express their care and concern?

Round and around my mind spun, and in the end I couldn't answer a single question. I tried to tell myself not to worry—after all, worry didn't help anyway—and then I would worry about the fact that I couldn't stop worrying! My obsessive mind refused to stop.

About the same time, I saw one of my patients and her husband standing in line at the local cineplex. I reached forward and tapped her left shoulder lightly, calling out her name. She whirled around, and looked at me with a blank stare. "Sue," I cried out. "It's me—Greg!"

"Greg?" She hesitated momentarily, unable to recognize me, the person who had sat face to face with her over a span of several weeks. "Oh…Greg. Wow! How…are…you?"

I responded the same way that most people do when asked that question; I lied. I hated lying, but it was one of those "good" types of lies, the kind you like to believe is protecting the other person, but is actually protecting yourself. Who wants to hear that you're scared shitless?

One other thing about lying; it's awfully contagious.

Back to Sue. "You look…good," she said in a halting voice. Even though I doubted her veracity, I gave her a free pass to the fair that day. After all, what the heck was she supposed to say? You look horrible? You look like death warmed over? You look just like my father did when he was in hospice?

I'm sure it was difficult for Sue to run into me that night, but at least she didn't have to guess whether or not I was still alive. It was a given that Katherine and I would run into someone we knew sooner or later, and I was afraid of the questions they might ask. As difficult as it was for me to go out in public, the thought of staying home and feeling sorry for myself was worse. It felt like solitary confinement on death row. I have always been a "people person," the kind of person that gets positive energy from being with others. My cancer didn't kill that desire. Other people put wild adventures on their bucket lists, such as walking across a bed of red-hot coals or traveling to far away places, but that just wasn't me. I wanted to spend every last remaining microsecond with the people I loved.

I made the tentative decision to return to work. I could tell that Katherine was afraid, but she went along with my plan as long as I agreed to start slowly and not exhaust myself.

I sent out a group email to my patients to inform them that I was coming back, and scheduled a few appointments. It felt good just to be able to talk briefly with them on the phone, and several mentioned how happy they were to hear that I was okay and able to work. Unlike with Sue, when they asked me how I was, I told them the truth. I was taking things one day at a time and was hopeful that I would continue to make progress.

One day at a time. Cancer had changed everything in my life, not the least of which was how I looked at the world. It was ironic that at the same time I was so frightened about losing my left eye, my vision actually improved. My intimacy with death revealed things to me that I had never seen before. Now I could clearly see that I lived in an amazing paradise. I saw thousands—maybe even a million billion—diamonds shimmering in the lake as the summer sun ascended into the sky. Suddenly I had become a very rich man.

The words spoken by one of the patients in the cardiac support group Katherine and I conducted came back to me: "My heart attack was the best thing that ever happened to me." He was an accountant by trade and, like most of the people in our group, he had a type A personality. After he was released from the cardiac care unit at the hospital, he spent several days on his back porch, listening to the birds sing. He spent so much time there that his wife thought he'd gone off the deep end. His heart attack was a shot across the bow and served as an awakening. Before his heart attack he was consumed with counting other people's money. After the attack he started counting the days he had left to live.

As compelling as his story was, it was chromosomally different from mine. He went on to live a low-fat, enlightened life, full of birdsong, whereas I was convinced that I was going to take my newly acquired wisdom to the grave. I berated myself. Why had I wasted so much of my life worrying about crap that either didn't happen or, in the long run, didn't matter?

My thoughts turned to Markel, my favorite character in Dostoevsky's *The Brothers Karamazov*. Markel was described as a "hot tempered and irritable" man whose personality changed dramatically after he fell ill from consumption. His family could not believe the change; his countenance became increasingly "glad" and "joyful" even as his physical condition deteriorated.

Markel went on to make several mystical pronouncements, such as his revelation that we all live in "paradise" but his family refused to believe it. His mother and the physician wouldn't buy into his metaphysical insights, concluding instead that Markel's illness had driven him mad.

But I agreed with Markel. I didn't know what would happen after I died, but for the time being, I too lived in paradise.

Unhappily, it was a realization that overwhelmed me. Instead of easing my mind, it only compounded my fears. I didn't want to leave paradise! If only I could have one more year...

THE NEXT MORNING the car keys felt different as I carefully inserted the silver one into the ignition. Everything about my drive to work was different that day: the blue water of the lake seemed bluer, the sound of the voices on the morning news program more resonant and full-bodied. Flow seemed as if she were on autopilot, cruising this way and that through the stretch of small inland lakes and into Traverse City. I swiped at tears as I drove by St. Patrick's church and remembered the frightful night when I fled into its sanctuary and begged God to save me.

Trying to keep some semblance of a routine, I went into the coffee shop across the street from my office. My favorite barista had apparently moved on, and an unfamiliar young woman with a prominent tattoo on her arm took my order for a half-caffeinated coffee. As I sat on the still-hard metal chair, reality hit and I realized how depleted I was and how much effort it took just to get into town. I looked down and fell into the blackness of my coffee. Maybe I should have stayed home after all.

"Here you go!" Suddenly a man's voice jolted me out of my reverie. It was my old coffeehouse nemesis, John. In his outstretched hand was a crumpled copy of the morning newspaper. There was no inquiry as to where I had been, no acknowledgment of my absence, no question asking what in the world had happened to me. To be fair, I didn't ask him what he had been up to either.

I thanked John for the newspaper and scanned the sports section and local news. Yet it was difficult for me to focus because I was distracted by the copy of the *Wall Street Journal* lying on the table next to me. April 1 flashed back through my mind, and my thoughts turned to my disease mate, Andy Martin. I wondered if he was still alive, but I was too afraid to look into it. I turned away from the *Journal*.

Like most things we dread, the morning turned out to go much better than expected. As I had predicted, my patients were very worried about me, but at the same time they seemed happy—relieved, anyway—to see me again. The depth of their compassion and sensitivity didn't surprise me. My experience over twenty-five years had convinced me that the vast majority of my patients were sensitive, flexible people who had been hurt by insensitive and rigid people.

To be honest, I was also relieved to see my patients. It was refreshing to focus on someone else's problems, and it was wonderful to feel like there was something I could still give. I needed to believe that my "work" on Earth was not finished yet; I was determined to keep at it. It was true I had crawled my way back to work, but there I was again, in my loyal leather chair that still needed polishing, listening to tales of abandonment, rejection, and heartache. I never revealed how badly I actually felt or shared any doubt that I would make it along the trail with them. They didn't need to hear it, and frankly, neither did I.

MEANWHILE, KATHERINE CONTINUED HER ALL-OUT assault on my cancer. We incorporated Libby's suggestions by fine-tuning my acupuncture treatments and adjusting the daily supplements. The cornerstone of Katherine's attack consisted of mega-doses of assorted vitamins and supplements. We spent hours stuffing hundreds of multi-colored pills of every size and color into tiny, plastic zip-lock pouches. Emerson was fascinated, and leaped in to help us in our "medicine factory." Fortunately, she was too young to understand the purpose and gravity of the situation.

Taking the pills became a defining part of my day. At the beginning and end of each day I swallowed a packet of mushroom extracts. As an appetizer before every meal, I ingested several proteolytic enzymes and anti-inflammatory herbs. I washed down high doses of vitamins with my main course. By the time I went to bed, I had ingested over 70 nonprescription pills!

I hated it. Some people love to fuss, but that's just not me. Sitting on the carpet, sorting out hundreds of piles of pills drove me crazier than I already was, if that was possible. But I would do whatever I had to…to live. Katherine was working around the clock to save my life, and she was my last hope. I tried to remain optimistic and keep pulling myself forward, but felt as though I were treading water—and I could barely keep my nose above the water line.

At the same time that I started working again, I also decided to return to the local gym, thinking it would help to jump-start my energy. But the climb up the two flights of steps to enter the muscle-bound world was incredibly difficult. Just a few short months ago I could run for miles on the treadmill. Those were the days when cancer was a bad disease that other people had. People like John, a popular local doctor who spent many of his last days on Earth in the same gym, trying anything he could to stay alive. I could tell he was sick—really sick. It was obvious the moment the previously buffed-out dude pushed through the gym doors. Cancer had reduced him to little more than a tall walking stick, and he struggled to keep his balance on the slowly revolving treadmill. It was hard to watch him stumble and flounder about. One day he stopped coming to the gym. Not long afterward his obituary appeared in the local paper.

Now it was my turn, my turn to…I stepped on the treadmill and began a slow, unsteady walk. As my steps began to feel a little more secure, my mind for some reason returned to that bizarre night at the cottage. There was Ali on the ropes, the fight well on the way to an expected conclusion. Yet he came back with a hell-bent fury to defeat Foreman. It seemed so auspicious at the time. I was beyond convinced that it was an omen.

Suddenly, I felt as if I were being commanded to act. Without thinking, I obliged. I clenched my fists and began shadow boxing, pummeling the damn tumor. I gave it everything I had! My left… my right…right again…left…and then I delivered a vicious knock-out punch that sent it into oblivion.

It was a great fantasy while it lasted, but it didn't take long for my fatigue to bring me back to reality. The cancer wasn't Foreman; it was cagier and much more lethal. And there was no way in hell I was Ali; I could barely keep slogging along for ten minutes on the treadmill! The reality was that I was more like John, a dying man trying to deny reality. I imagined what other people in the gym must have thought when they looked at me: a razor-thin dude with wisps of white hair, violently shaking his fists at the sky. It was so obvious; I was one very sick man.

NOTHING SEEMED TO BE WORKING. The swelling in my face refused to obey my wishes and go away. I was convinced that the cancer was marching through my body. Fear engulfed me. Four months had passed since my initial diagnosis, and there was still no sign that I was getting any better. Still, Katherine and I kept our promise to each other to keep up our assault on the tumor.

Truth be told, I was in big trouble, and I couldn't hang on much longer. It was incredibly difficult to make it through each day. I was unbelievably anxious and had zero appetite. What was the point of putting us all through this stuff if it wasn't working? I looked up from my plate of food and saw Emerson, sitting happily in her chair, chatting away about something or the other, and Katherine, half listening and trying hard to refrain from telling me to eat.

The fight had exhausted me and worn down my defenses. It had been sixteen weeks of unremitting hell, and I was ready to give up. My psychic wall caved in, and a deep depression washed over me.

My recurring nightmare returned to haunt me that night:

I'm on the jet. This time the jet was barely above ground, flying between tall buildings in a large city. It was clear that we were not going to make it to the airport and that the plane would crash. The jet landed on a busy street and rolled to a stop. I climbed out of the window onto the wing, then jumped from the wing to the ground. I ran around, screaming, trying to find a phone so I could let everyone know that I was okay.

The next thing I knew Katherine was grabbing me and trying to wake me. She told me I had been shouting out for help and offered me great comfort as I described the nightmare to her.

Something inside me was dying. The optimism that had served others and me so well was gone. I believed my situation was hopeless, and like many depressed men, I became increasingly irritable. Everything and everybody was wrong. Despair ruled my consciousness and negativity was the order of the day. I'm ashamed to admit that I went so far as to bite the devoted hand that was trying to feed me, and Katherine felt the sting. Of course my ungratefulness made me feel that much worse about myself.

KATHERINE

THINGS REMAINED THE SAME and that sameness was an unwelcome state of being. Our lives were dominated by fear, death, illness, and anxiety. I rejected the oncologists' "wait and see" attitude. Maybe Greg had begun to plateau and, admittedly, he wasn't on the horrifying downward spiral we had lived through in July, but he was so far from any meaningful state of health that it was impossible for me to sit back and wait. Wait for what? Little did I know the sameness and waiting were just a resting place. We were being pulled towards something far greater…a crossroads that demanded we make a choice.

Greg awoke at 4:30 a.m., desperate and unable to breathe. Once his racing heart began to slow, he snapped on the bedside light. He was filled with frustration and refused to talk or allow me to hold him. Instead, he dressed and left the house. Perhaps his abrupt departure was an act of defiance toward his vulnerability. I remained awake in the unsettled predawn darkness and slowly found my way to my desk and my own process with my pen. There was comfort there, as my own chaotic state shifted into the present moment.

I listened to the cool steady rain and hoped it would be a soaking one that lasted all day. I thought of small, immediate things. Too bad I hadn't gotten Emerson a raincoat—well, an umbrella would do. The rain soothed me and I imagined the newest members of my garden were equally comforted: my scarlet Lucifer, leafy coral-bells, and the purple monarda. But as the rain drummed on the roof, the comfort morphed into exhaustion and wrapped around me like a heavy cloak.

I reflected upon how far I had come. I had found the building, the architect, the renovation team, the accountant, lawyer, and potential staff. I had almost finished my letter of explanation to my patients, but stopped when the fear and apprehension returned. I could not agree to a closing date or lift my pen to sign the purchase agreement. I needed to make a decision. It occurred to me I had been here before.

My mind drifted to a distant winter when Greg and I traveled to Maui on a retreat. It was a sunny morning, and we eagerly set out on a hike through the tropical rainforest near Hana to the Seven Sacred Pools. After an hour or so we reached a pristine waterfall and stood beside the 700-foot canyon walls covered with ferns and wild impatiens. We yelped in delight as the rain-fed waterfall splashed our hatless heads and sweaty bodies. Refreshed, we began our descent, crossing rocky gulches and waterless stream beds.

As we hiked through majestic bamboo forests and listened to the melodic sounds of the bamboo trunks tapping against one another, I could hear people in the distance hooting and hollering. We chased their excited cries and laughter through the forest and finally discovered the source of the commotion. An enthusiastic group of Australians were jumping off a cliff ledge into a pool of water 30 feet below. As we drew nearer, I felt a magnetic pull to join in. The prospect was at once exhilarating and frightening. After watching for fifteen minutes, it was my turn to jump. I backed away. I had more than second thoughts, and said dismissively to Greg, "I don't need to do this! It's not that important to me!"

Despite the bravado of my words, we both knew that I was afraid. It was clear I wanted to jump into the crystalline blue water in the heat of the day, but my mind conjured up images of disaster and I clung to the illusion of security. *Come back! Don't do it!* I stood there for a few minutes that seemed like hours, contemplating the leap of faith. Now here I was years later, wanting to jump.

Did I have the courage to leap into a new practice? Now of all times? Greg seemed to have aged several decades after the dual assault of chemo and radiation; he'd become an old man overnight. He struggled with congestion, exhaustion, and defeat. I feared the cancer was reestablishing itself, and that I would soon be dealing with the unthinkable—I soon would be a widow. How could I go on without him? Who would help me raise Emerson?

In Hawaii I'd stood on a ledge of warm grey stone, looking down at the pool of cool water beckoning me. I couldn't make myself jump. And I couldn't take on the $400,000 debt and emotional investment when Greg's health was still so tenuous and our paths so uncertain.

Everything seemed up for grabs. I questioned whether I should even continue to practice medicine. I wondered if I really had what it took to be a healer. Honestly, I didn't even know what the term meant anymore. I wasn't convinced about the power of any kind of medicine. Traditional? Alternative? I had serious misgivings about all of it. Did any of it really help?

I placed the cap on my pen, pushed back my chair, bundled up Emerson and the umbrella. I drove us to school and work with my teeth digging into my lower lip. As the rain splattered on my windshield, I vowed to love the questions, even though they tasted so bitter in my mouth.

What was my destiny?

The windshield wipers pounded.

To support and love people on their life journey, my heart pounded its answer.

May it be a healing experience for us all.

22.

MASTER LEE

KATHERINE

AT THE END OF THE MONTH, Brenin packed up and flew to Portland, Oregon, to begin his life at Reed College. At least he was on the same continent this time, although still over 3,000 miles away. I wouldn't see him again until Christmas break—unless tragedy called him home sooner.

The heat and vitality of summer retreated into the last days of August. Vibrant greens turned to burnished yellows. The waters of Duck Lake grew colder as the nights dipped into the 50s. Each day I forced myself to go for one last swim in the grey-green waters that surged at the dock. Geese began their southward migration. Like the waves, we were always in motion with errands, work, and parenting.

Greg continued to work part-time and to care for Emerson while I worked at my office and the hospital. He would nap while she napped; he was forever tired and his appetite was still tenuous. He put a temporary moratorium on taking any supplements, saying he just needed a break. I had to admit that I did too. It forced me to quit distracting myself with all the doing and open my eyes to what was really happening. The sameness had become a slow poison. I stopped pretending that things were fine, and reality spilled out. Greg was desperately ill.

I reached out to one of my medical school colleagues. David had risen to national prominence as a highly respected neurologist with expertise in alternative and complementary therapies. His approach was controversial, though grounded in scientific principles and peer-reviewed research. I trusted and respected him. Late one Friday afternoon, I called him on the phone and asked his advice about Greg. David cared for people who made life and death decisions on a daily basis. I discussed the nutritional testing and other approaches that we were contemplating. After several minutes, he kindly interrupted me and said emphatically, "What Greg needs to do is to go see Master Lee. He is a remarkable man with great experience, and he will be of help to you now." David's conviction and confidence filled the void that I felt.

Since the first month of Greg's diagnosis, I had been inundated with emails and anecdotal reports of cancer cures from well-meaning friends and strangers. Everyone had a recommendation on how to treat cancer. I would wade through the information and scratch my head: they had to be kidding! Some advice made no sense at all, and others twisted science to fit their unfounded conclusions.

I could see how easily people like us, desperate and afraid, could grasp at mirages of cure and promises of survival. I knew there was a thin line between cutting-edge ideas and wishful interpretations. I wanted to work with individuals who had a credible track record, someone who would review the treatment I had pieced together and tell us what to alter or add. We needed someone to help us execute a plan for the months ahead that included diet, a daily routine, as well as supplements, herbs, and acupuncture.

I began investigating Master Lee and his New Life Center located in the Jamaica Plains neighborhood of Boston. Over the course of several days, I had conversations with the staff and Master Lee himself. The Center was a residential program for patients with life-threatening diseases, primarily cancer. Unfortunately, the Center was closed as they were between sessions, but as we talked, they agreed to accommodate our small family. Since we were coming off-cycle, we would all be able to live at the Center while Greg received his treatments by Master Lee and the ancillary staff. Greg was hesitant, but we said good-bye to our recent dream of spending a last week of summer at a small cottage on Lake Michigan. We packed our bags for the big city of Boston.

GREG

KATHERINE REFUSED TO GIVE UP. When she told me she wanted me to go to an acupuncture center run by some Korean guy with the name "Master Lee," my newly developed cynicism got the best of both of us. Master Lee? The New Life Center? Are you kidding me? What kind of acupuncture can he do that you can't?

Like many cynics, I was long on assumptions and prejudice and short on facts and experience. Of course, I wasn't about to let reality get in my way, and I continued to spout off to Katherine. I dug in my heels. No way was I going! It was stupid! Why do we have to go? I was a little kid again, not wanting to go to the doctor and get a shot. I was so sick and tired of being so sick and tired!

Well, the next thing I knew we were packing our bags for the trip to Boston. While Katherine gave me plenty of space to be in my pissy mood, she insisted that we give the center a try. At the end of the day I surrendered. Once again, I remembered our vow to each other in the conference room at the Cancer Center: we would do anything and everything. Going to see Master Lee fell squarely into that category.

KATHERINE

AS OUR PLANE TOUCHED DOWN at Logan Airport I reached over and kissed Emerson's smiling face and squeezed Greg's hand. Immediately I sensed his reluctance as he braced himself once more for the unknown. Oddly, I felt we were going exactly where we needed to; yet my analytical mind had no idea where that was. Call it my sixth sense. I had to have the courage to follow it…for both of us.

My older sister, Joan, and her husband Frank met us once we cleared security. It was wonderful to see her familiar face and hear her loud, quirky laugh assert itself over the airport commotion. For a moment, I almost believed we were on vacation, like so many other passengers that August day. My wishful thinking disappeared as we all hugged and I saw my husband's withered body in their arms.

It came like this, unexpected, without bidding. Like when he put his arms around me and I held his delicate frame against my body. It was in these moments that I prayed with earnest: *Show me the way. Let my heart not be deceived by this temporary illusion. Lift our love upward so that we may be of service and an inspiration to others.* Greg's illness had broken my heart wide open.

The devastation lifted just as quickly as it came. I shifted my focus to our reunion with loved ones. We picked up our bags, shouldered our backpacks, and held each other's hands. We chatted cheerfully and walked through the crowded airport.

We spent the weekend with Joan and Frank on Cape Cod. They had a modest motor home that was permanently parked in Dennis Port just outside of South Yarmouth. Joan and Frank slept in their friend's nearby home, so we could have the luxury of the 150-square-foot space to ourselves. We swam every day in the salty waters of the Atlantic. Initially, Emerson held onto us for dear life, but she gradually relaxed into the buoyancy of the gentle waves. We ate delicious meals of fresh crab and raw oysters. During quiet moments, we shared the meaningful details of our past months.

The nights were still, and we could hear muffled traffic on the small road that separated us from the waters of Nantucket Sound. Greg's sleep was fitful. He woke up often. Times like this tried my patience. I wanted to sleep so badly, and just when I was in the deepest stages, his cries would yank me back. Not again! I wanted to pull the pillow over my head. Of course, part of me resented it, and the other part understood he was fighting for his life. Like a mother with a sick child, I would find my way to compassion and rise to the demands of otherness.

I found a new ritual that sometimes worked to ease his fitful body back to sleep. I rubbed his feet with a mild hormone cream. I knew from my endocrinology studies that progesterone provided a calming hormone that helped with anxiety, insomnia, and irritability. It was most often prescribed to women for PMS and menstrual irregularity, but men needed it too, in smaller amounts. In both sexes, progesterone is sidetracked during a crisis into making the stress hormone, cortisol, instead of performing its usual calming function. This singular phenomenon is referred to as the "cortisol steal." The cream rubbed into Greg's skin traveled into his bloodstream and offered additional progesterone to soothe his frayed psyche. It worked 75 percent of the time, and thankfully it did that night.

After the respite of the long weekend, we packed and began the Sunday morning drive into Boston. Joan cruised the merging highways with their increasing complexity and innumerable exit ramps until she found the one for Jamaica Plains. She navigated the city's maze of one-way roads until she found the tree-lined streets with their well-groomed Victorian houses. She came to a slow stop on Harris Street, and parked in front of a light yellow, blue-shuttered, two-story house. A small sign on the porch read, "The New Life Center." We had arrived.

We piled out of the car and paused in the quiet of Sunday morning. A few birds rustled in the hedge. We left our bags in the car and trekked up the stairs to the front porch. A small sign read "Please Enter," and the door jingled as we stepped through it into a large porch with filtered light. Slippers of all sizes sat in a basket next to a bench. We stood suspended in the quiet of the foyer for several minutes until a young Korean woman entered. She shuffled quietly in her slippers across the wooden floor to greet us. Her silky black hair was drawn smoothly into a ponytail, revealing her lovely face with a full smile and kind eyes.

"Hello, welcome to the New Life Center. My name is Suni. May I help you?"

We explained that we were the expected visitors, and she showed us upstairs to our room. It was simple and clean with high ceilings and windows that opened onto the lush, green-leafed trees outside. There was a dresser, a closet, and two double beds. A small mattress lay on the floor. I put down my suitcase and smiled at our good fortune.

Suni invited us to have lunch, and extended the offering to Joan and Frank. They agreed to join us before heading home to their other life in North Attleboro. We were ushered downstairs into a dining room with low tables and small cushions. A serving table was lined with several mysterious dishes. A large salad bowl was filled with cooked green leaves that we later learned was Korean seaweed. There was also stewed yellow curried chicken, a vegetable dish with okra and peas, rice, and tea. We cautiously filled our plates and sat on the cushioned floor. We raised our chopsticks and tasted this new food. I thought it was delicious and felt nourishing: Emerson and Greg weren't so sure. Joan and Frank found all of it so interesting and beamed while nodding their heads at us from across the intimate table. We began to settle into our new home for the week.

GREG

JOAN AND FRANK WERE THEIR USUAL loving and caring selves, and both were optimistic that I was going to "beat" the cancer. It was refreshing to be with them, and helpful to focus on someone other than myself. They had gone through tough times of their own: Joan with her emotional sequela from past difficult marriages, Frank with painful complications following a botched hip surgery.

Just as we were about to say adios to Frank, he handed me a small package and told me that it was something he and Joan wanted me to have. I opened the gift, and saw that it was the bottom half of a Celtic cross Katherine and I had purchased for them during a poetry retreat in Ireland. Frank revealed that he and Joan were going to keep the top half of the cross. They believed that one day I would defeat the cancer, return to the Cape, and claim the missing half. I choked back my tears wanting it to be true! I couldn't imagine such a possibility. I didn't have any doubts, however, about Frank and Joan's powerful love and compassion.

The magic spell of the Cape quickly dissipated as we joined the thousands of other refugees returning to the megalopolis. We arrived at the New Life Center in Jamaica Plains late Sunday afternoon. I didn't like the name of the clinic. New Life? I wasn't interested in a "new life" at all: I wanted my old life back! The one where I lived in a small town with my perfect little family. The one where Katherine and I helped a few people here and there, and enjoyed our unpretentious lives. It may not have been the good life for other people, but it was the one we cherished. It was ours, and it was fast disappearing.

The New Life Center was a residential treatment facility with sleeping quarters located on the second floor. The treatment rooms, staff offices, and outpatient waiting area were located on the first level, and the dining area in the basement. We were informed that Master Lee and his family lived in the back section of the building.

The staff member politely explained the schedule, the centerpiece of which was acupuncture treatments and lectures to be given by Master Lee. The three daily meals of Korean food would be served buffet-style. There were additional services that we could add a la carte, such as therapeutic massage and consultations about herbs and supplements. She led us to our room.

Once the staff member excused herself, we unpacked our bags and set up camp. As I thumbed through the package of material, I noticed a shiny white button about the size of a half dollar coin. "New Life Center" was proudly imprinted in cornflower blue writing on the top of the coin, and on the bottom were the words, "We Have Hope."

Hope. The four-letter word that the oncologists at the Cancer Center had been so reluctant to utter, the word that we were so hungry to hear! There it was, in bold print, right in front of me, the motto of Master Lee's clinic! They not only had hope, they were proud of it—so proud that they displayed it, like a sign on a motel trumpeting that the rooms have Wi-Fi. So they had hope. As I switched off the bedside light, I had a flicker of hope that Master Lee could help me.

KATHERINE

WE SETTLED INTO THE OLD HOUSE and unpacked our small bags. Emerson lined her stuffed animals and art supplies along the deep windowsills. We set out to explore the neighborhood and discovered a modest street lined with an assortment of shops. Everything was closed that Sunday, with the exception of the mom and pop corner market. Emerson was captivated by a small toy store, and we lingered for half an hour looking at all the bright, cheerful objects in the window. Backtracking, we headed south past Victorian houses with their black iron gates to the small park beside the Amtrak station. The swings, climbing structures, and benches provided refuge for the afternoon. We played together, and intermittently cast out greetings to the few visitors who wandered by. It was a quintessential Sunday afternoon and time drifted surreally.

Monday morning arrived and the New Life Center came alive with…well, new life. Master Lee had a busy schedule filled with patients from the Boston area who traveled by subway, bus, and even foot to see him. Today Greg was one of them. The examination and treatment area was located in a large room with five or six cots separated by retractable curtains that provided a small measure of privacy. We could overhear conversations between Master Lee and the patient on the other side of the curtain. Thankfully, the voices were muffled. Simple greetings and yes and no replies were about all I could make out, and only if I really strained, which I didn't.

The curtain slid open and Master Lee stood before us. He was diminutive in stature, standing only an inch or two above my five-foot-three-inch frame. His skin was golden amber and his hair shocking white. His eyebrows, still black, accented his eyes with their aging sparkle. His face was wide, with a half smile that showed his strong teeth. He took my hands in both of his and gave a bow with the downward tilt of his head. He spoke about Dr. Perlmutter with familiarity and fondness.

After Master Lee's warm welcome, he turned his attention to Greg and bowed his head again. He proceeded to look at him with a direct, straight-on gaze. Words flew from his mouth, chopped and to the point. "You sick? Where?"

Greg pointed to his left cheek and said, equally simply, "Here. Sinus cancer."

"Lie down. Please." Greg unfurled himself like a sail with no wind. "Now show me tongue." He stared for several minutes at Greg's raw, red tongue. Then he placed the fingers of both his hands on Greg's upturned wrists. Again, a long pause followed. His hands moved to Greg's abdomen, and he palpated both sides carefully and intently. Master Lee turned to me and waved me over to his side.

"See kidney weaker on this side. Not balanced with heart."

To him, his observation was so clear and diagnostic; to me, it was obscure and confusing. I could feel that one quadrant of Greg's belly was more tense than the other side. But what did it mean? Before I could ask, he returned his laser-like focus to Greg.

"You have pain?" he queried.

Greg offered back, "No pain, but fullness here." His left hand rose again to his left cheek.

"Tell me when fullness gone!" Master Lee directed. He quickly placed several acupuncture needles into Greg's ankle and right outer calf, and began to rotate the needles vigorously.

"Awwwh!" Greg yelped.

"Change? No 'awwh.' Tell me when fullness gone!" He moved quickly to the other side of Greg's body and placed another needle in his left hand.

"Tell me when change!" Dr. Lee said. He continued to move like a musician around Greg's body, intent on tuning it to some vibration that I could not hear. I imagined each needle accessing a different chord, and each turn of the needle able to raise or lower the pitch. He commanded that Greg not distract himself with the discomfort, but to focus on his awareness of the sinus fullness.

After five or more minutes of this dance between them, Greg murmured, "It's better. Yes, it's better."

Master Lee resumed his stationary posture, coming to stand silently beside Greg. "This good. Yes?" He spoke in Korean to his assistant, who had entered the curtained cloister. She wrote down the specific points and other details, which I failed to comprehend. I had been more absorbed with the exchange of energy and the dance between Greg and Master Lee. I thought of my own one-year training in acupuncture through UCLA. Americans typically object to discomfort or pain from the treatment, whereas people in the East desire stronger treatments that they believe are more effective. I knew Greg would agree that Master Lee's aggressive approach was much different from mine.

"I see you tomorrow," Master Lee announced. He moved through the curtain, leaving Greg to rest with the needles in place. Ten minutes later the assistant slid them out. I helped Greg off the cot and scooped up a wide-eyed Emerson.

So the treatment had begun. As important as it might be for Greg, I realized in a vague, intuitive sort of way that it would be equally therapeutic for me.

GREG

WE CLIMBED OUT OF THE SACK EARLY that Monday morning and made our way down a maze of stairways to breakfast, Korean style. There were no cereal boxes with doped up athletes on their covers, no short stacks of pancakes smothered in sugar-laden syrup. Instead there was rice—lots and lots of small perfectly sculpted mounds of white rice. There were several serving trays full of colorful combinations of vegetables and tofu. This was not a breakfast of champions; this was a breakfast for the survivors.

I was so thankful that Emerson ate what was offered without complaint or tantrum. She was no stranger to rice and vegetables. Katherine and I had agreed from the start we were going to feed Emerson the same food we ate. So when she was ready for solid food, we introduced her to the world of veggies. She was a frequent companion on my shopping trips to the local food co-op where she loved to share a tempeh Rueben sandwich with me for lunch.

After breakfast, we made our way up to the main floor and to a treatment room where I was directed to hop up on one of the three treatment tables. Thin, white cloth curtains hung on metal rods in an effort to create a semblance of privacy between the tables. It was clear that other patients would be able to listen in on everything that happened to me. It felt like being in a dentist office where you can hear the dentist drilling away on the poor soul in the next room.

The curtain pulled back and Master Lee walked in. He reached out to us with both of his small hands and welcomed us to the Center. His slender body was neatly dressed in khaki pants, and a checked short-sleeve shirt. There was a large bald spot on the top of his head that evenly separated two patches of white hair. His posture and speech exuded confidence, without the arrogance that often accompanies it.

Master Lee wasted no time on social niceties; he was all business. He shot several questions at me in broken English: "What bothering you? Pain? Where pain? There? Here? Hurt bad?" I did the best I could to keep up with his rapid-fire questioning, and it was immediately obvious that he was not interested in any elaborations or qualifications. There was no room for maybes in this yes or no, black and white interview.

Master Lee began to stick needles in various places all over my body. I was used to Katherine's acupuncture treatments, but Master Lee's way of doing things was a whole different story. The needles felt huge, and he wasn't shy about sticking them in. Once the needle was in, he twisted and turned it in different directions while asking if I had more or less pain.

It hurt like hell, so much so that I let out a yelp. Master Lee's small, dark eyes looked down at me. "You not dying!" he declared in an uncharacteristically loud voice. My body thought otherwise, however, and I continued to recoil from the incoming needles. "You not dying!" he repeated, much louder this time, as if I hadn't heard him the first time. Not dying? I didn't know what he was talking about. Was he talking about the cancer, or was he trying to get me to stop complaining?

He twisted and turned the needles this way, that way, up, down. Once he was satisfied with the placement, he left my bedside and closed the cloth curtain behind him. A few minutes later I heard him bring another patient into the room, followed by the sound of curtains swishing along a metal rod. I could listen to every word of their conversation. My body stiffened in sympathy as I anticipated the needles being jammed into the patient and the screaming that would surely follow, but none came. I didn't know what that patient felt, if anything, but I decided it was going to be one long week.

KATHERINE

GREG HOVERED ABOUT IN A STATE OF IRRITABILITY and anxiety. There we were, in a place with no distractions from his illness. Paradoxically, instead of the focus being beneficial, the treatments and the constant attention to his deteriorated state were challenging for him. I sensed he just wanted to get on with his life and leave the Center.

In contrast, I found both the house and the routine to be calming and restorative. The three of us were together, and we were being cared for by a loving family. I saw a true goodness in all of it, regardless of the imperfections. The slower pace soothed my exhausted, frayed nerves. Suni's food was delicious, and I was grateful not to be the one doing all the shopping, cooking, and cleaning. I knew Greg and little Emerson wanted more variety, but my ears were impervious to their complaints. Too bad, I thought. They would surely find some way to survive.

Each day was a gift to me. The mornings were luxurious, and I would awaken in the spacious, high-ceilinged room with Emerson asleep beside me on the floor. More often than not, Greg had already dressed and gone out for a walk. I opened the window for the fresh air and soft, filtered light that would fall on me as I stretched out on the unmade bed. I filled the unclaimed moments with writing, thinking, and pondering my dreams.

I was especially grateful to have someone else care for Greg. Their attentiveness and treatments lifted a huge weight from my shoulders. Master Lee and his family allowed me to step away from Greg's pain and suffering in a way I had not been able to for many months. I still trembled when I thought back to that first day of April and the exhausting battle we'd fought relentlessly every minute of every day since. I listened half-heartedly as Greg complained about the costs of the extra treatments at the New Life Center. I couldn't put a price tag on them. Now that we were there, I suspended my critical mind and vigilance. I invited the experience to have its way with us.

Each day after Master Lee's treatment, Greg was encouraged to have one additional therapy. The first was for a posture evaluation and Korean bodywork. Dr. Lee's younger brother Mark was the therapist, and well versed in many other therapeutic modalities including massage, herbalism, and movement therapies, specifically yoga and tai chi.

His evaluation of Greg's posture revealed nothing new, yet reinforced what other therapists had pointed out previously. He had the habit of forward thrusting his head, which shortened and flexed his neck. This caused the rounding of his shoulders and collapsing of his chest, which constricted both his breath and blood flow to his head. Mark worked with Greg to help him correct this tendency, and showed him how it expanded his breathing and circulation. The extra oxygen was good for his overall health, plus it slowed the growth of cancer, which thrives on low-oxygen or anaerobic states. Interestingly, over the ensuing years Mark's belief has been validated. Low-oxygen states are a big player in what initiates and promotes cancer.[1]

Greg seemed unmoved by the evaluation and took it like his mother scolding him to stand up straight. Sure, it might be easy for someone else to see, but not so simple for the person looking out from his or her own body, with familiar patterns so tied into emotional memory.

The next morning Greg had a massage. I was allowed to be there by his side, and discovered it to be quite different from Western massage. There was attention to Greg's tight muscles and areas of restriction, but focus was also given to increasing blood flow. The ultimate goal was to get stagnation moving and allow the qi (life force) to flow and toxins to be removed. A unique technique called cupping was used. A dozen or more glass cups, about the size of small juice glasses, were placed on Greg's back from neck to sacrum on either side of his spine. The cups were then connected to a motorized device that extracted the air out of them so that they attached themselves with suction. Slowly the skin was sucked into each cup and allowed to remain there for ten or more minutes. As if he were in the arms of an octopus, Greg's skin turned bright red in a majority of the sites. According to Mark's assessment, this engorgement of blood was confirmation that stagnation was present. To my surprise, Greg found it very relaxing and fell asleep. When it was over I had to nudge him back to wakefulness. When he mentioned the extra cost, I shrugged my shoulders and told him he was worth every penny.

The next day Mark, the herbalist, created a medicinal tea for Greg to drink three times a day. I visited Mark in his basement "kitchen." It was a large laboratory, immaculately clean, with steel tables and shelves from floor to ceiling filled with containers of herbs. He would concoct a new brew every few days for Greg under the direction of Master Lee. The herbs were soaked for hours in a vat

1   http://www.ncbi.nlm.nih.gov/pubmed/21606941

that resembled a huge pressure cooker, then slowly simmered. After the tea cooled, it was divided into servings and packaged in pressure-sealed Baggies. I found the technique and precision inspiring. I understood the basic goals of the herbs—to build qi and blood, as well as to calm disturbed shen (spirit).

During our third night at the center, Greg was tormented with anxiety and panic. We phoned Master Lee and asked for help, even though it was after midnight. He came immediately to our small room and talked with us. "We must watch ourselves," Master Lee said. "Watch your thoughts, your mind. It is for you to discover your attachments. What are you running towards? What are you running from—the fears and repressions? Stop the running! Stop the thinking!" He encouraged us once more, "We must all do our homework!" He took Greg in his arms, held him, and told him he loved him. Somehow Greg was able to grab the reins of his runaway stagecoach and find his way to sleep.

The next morning I contemplated Master Lee's instructions. What were our attachments? What were we running toward? Success, bright things in the toy shop window, acceptance from some great authority?

What were we running from? What were we afraid of? Suffering, bowls of seaweed salad, needles, a shriveled body, death? All of it was dancing, forever changing, right in front of us. It was as if we were in a hall of mirrors, running from some and toward others, yet never sure which way we were ultimately headed. Master Lee's instructions were so simple. Stop the dance and just be with what was. Be where we were. Simple—but not easy.

DURING OUR STAY we had a medical consultation with Master Lee's son, Dr. Lee, who was a Western trained internist. The three of us reviewed Greg's diagnosis, lab reports, and treatment regimen.

I had carefully written down all the treatments Greg had received, and what he continued to take and do.

We reviewed his blood work and cell analysis. Greg had a mild anemia, and decreased white cell and killer cells. These were common side effects of radiation, and Western medicine had little to offer him. The Eastern medical interpretation was that Greg needed herbs to support blood production and strengthen digestion, which ultimately encouraged blood formation. In addition to the Chinese herbs and blood tonics, Dr. Lee recommended digestive enzymes, including hydrochloric acid with each meal. He then broached the issue of removing the heavy metals present in Greg's mercury amalgam fillings. He was concerned the mercury could leach from Greg's mouth into his body and weaken his immunity. They were so close to the area of the cancer that Dr. Lee felt there could be some connection. I had considered this before, but had been hesitant to encourage Greg to undergo another painful, invasive treatment until he was stronger. Dr. Lee encouraged us to find a qualified dentist and begin the process immediately. He also presented ways to strengthen his immune cells with medicinal mushrooms.

The more we talked and reviewed the last five months, the more I felt validated for all the efforts and choices we'd made, including the decisions to undergo chemo and radiation. I respected Dr. Lee, and he supported the months of research that I had done. Libby had been helpful, and I appreciated her input, but Dr. Lee was the first physician who valued and understood what we had done, making only minor adjustments and refinements to the treatment plan.

When we left the consultation room, my head was spinning with new ideas and questions. I was eager to take Dr. Lee's recommendations home and implement them. The Center did offer hope after all!

Greg took my hand and invited me to take off for the afternoon. I agreed, and suggested we take a picnic to the nearby arboretum.

He had a bigger idea. He wanted to strike out for an adventure in the city of Boston. He longed not to be a patient anymore. He just wanted to be my husband and Emerson's father. His request, so sincere, watered my love for him with its profound sweetness. How could I resist?

As we sat on the tattered seats of the public transit bus I pleaded with Greg to accept Master Lee's challenge and to be half as curious about his inner world as he was in the outer. Hadn't he gone through the chemo and radiation without a complaint? Now he balked at so much—the tea, the supplements, the treatments. Why? Finally, I told myself to put the bone down and to look at my own attachments. I chided myself, "You take the challenge. Let the path and its teachings unfold."

We settled back against the bus seat and held hands. I noticed that we were already in the bustling city. It was still summertime. Emerson swung her legs as she sat happily between us. We gave a small tug on the overhead cord to signal the driver that we wanted to get off at the Boston Public Garden exit. We strolled in the park under the sycamore tree canopy until we reached a small pond with a dozen or more swan boats. We rented a boat and paddled beside the rhododendrons, amidst the lily pads. Emerson leaned over the boat's edge and peered into the dark waters. The swish of the paddles as they turned under the boat murmured to me, "Love and support each other. Again and again. Each moment. Choose again."

That night I dreamt that I was on a long bicycle trip and stopped along the roadside to examine my front tire. Much to my dismay, I saw that it was flat. Not now! I was in the middle of an elaborate project in which I was building a miniature village with a multitude of tiny bridges. It seemed vitally important, even though it was a small version of the real thing.

I opened my eyes and lingered in the way station between the dream and my life. I didn't need psychoanalysis to figure it out. I was depleted, but I still had my vision; I needed to be resuscitated, or inspired, and begin to build the larger version of the miniature.

My memory drifted back to a conversation I'd had some twenty years earlier. I was in my third year of family medicine residency training in Seattle, Washington. My advisor met with me to evaluate my performance on the toughest assignment of my training.

During that time I was in charge of some of the sickest patients in the hospital, including patients in the Intensive Care Unit as well as those who were admitted through the Emergency Room. I was on call every three nights, and it was rare if I got an hour or two of sleep. The next morning I would have to discuss all of the admissions that had occurred the previous night to a roomful of senior physicians.

The rest of the doctors were well-rested and meticulously dressed for the day whereas I scrambled to find a moment to splash water on my face, brush my teeth, and comb my hair. Then the grueling ordeal would begin. I was expected to describe each patient in full detail, including their life history and present illness, with all the pertinent laboratory and physical findings, then conclude with my diagnosis and management. I had to do all of this from memory, in just three to five minutes per patient. The doctors would then ask for additional details and critique all of my decisions. I would feel sick and shaky each morning as I entered the conference room, and would stumble out relieved that the patients and I had survived. One night, when I had been especially challenged with several patients near death, my senior resident took me aside and said, "Why didn't you call me in?" I looked him in the eye and said to my defense, "Nobody died!" To put it lightly, I was being pushed to my limit physically, intellectually, and emotionally.

I remembered clearly how my advisor looked at me over his bifocals and said gently, "Katherine, you have competence. What you need is confidence!"

Damn it! How could I still have the same issues twenty years later? Yet, somehow, in this unusual place I was discovering my confidence. I was facing the most difficult medical case of my life and pioneering my own power of healing. That morning I knew the right way for me was to honor my courage! Celebrate my open heart and all that I did know! It had nothing to do with the future or what other physicians thought. I had found a way that allowed me to be humble and yet empowered.

The day before, Master Lee had said to me, "Don't watch your husband. Watch yourself!" He continued, "No judgments, no criticism. Just observe." He was dead right. I was forever watching Greg, scanning his face, his posture, and his moods; always looking for signs of health or illness. I vowed right then to see his presence, his dignity, his life force, and to honor and support it. I let everything go. I put the diagnosis of cancer behind us and believed in his healing.

In that moment, I returned to that ledge over the clear blue Hawaiian pond. In my mind I finally was able to let go. I jumped. Freedom surged through the free fall of my body, and the tropical air rushed through my hair as I plunged into the delicious coolness. It was time to go home.

GREG

THE ACUPUNCTURE TREATMENTS at the Center were followed in the afternoon by pep-talky lectures from Master Lee about the mind-body connection and the nature of consciousness. Katherine recalls the talks as inspirational, but I can't tell you a thing about them. I couldn't focus; my mind was anywhere but there.

My anxiety continued to climb and reach new heights, like the swell of waves building on the ocean during a hurricane. I had no idea why I felt so panicky, but I believe that on an unconscious level I sensed my time running out. Five months had passed since my diagnosis, and I was scheduled to have the tell-all PET scan and MRI in five, short weeks. We would soon find out how far the cancer had advanced and how much longer I had to live.

I felt trapped. I was at my wit's end trying to find a way out, but there was none. I was becoming more and more restless, and Master Lee's Center felt claustrophobic. I needed to find some escape, no matter how small, so I started to take walks each morning down into the business district of Jamaica Plains with its variety of small shops and restaurants.

Emerson and Katherine often meandered down the avenue with me, and we would pause and look in the windows of the various storefronts. During one of our walks, Emerson became very excited when she found a pink calculator in the shape of a cat's face. We agreed to get it for her at the end of the week, provided she continued to be a big girl. Emerson was thrilled by her discovery, and I was happy for her until I imagined Katherine, a widow, telling her how the daddy she used to have bought the kitty cat calculator for her.

I hated the Korean breakfasts. I could handle the nutritious, well-prepared food for lunch and dinner, no problem, but for breakfast? No way. That's where I drew the line in the sand. On one of my forays into the business district, I spied a small, hole-in-the wall bakery; the kind with big glass cases stuffed with rows and rows of sugar-glazed donuts, creamy Long Johns, and fat Bismarcks full of colorful jelly. The next morning, I began my daily ritual of sneaking off to the bakery to eat a bagel slathered in cream cheese. I had been such a good boy for weeks on end, doing everything anyone asked of me. The lightly toasted, everything bagel (yes, it had butter on it too) wasn't what the doctor ordered, but it was great for my mental health. Freedom never tasted so good!

I didn't hesitate to confess my dietary sin to Katherine; in fact, I admit I took no small amount of self-satisfaction telling her about my defiant behavior. It's bizarre to think that my last stand might have been eating a bagel at a bakery, but there I was, enjoying every bite. My only complaint was that the bakery didn't have any lox. Katherine never once raised an objection to my daily transgression. She seemed relieved that I was interested in eating anything.

Our week at the New Life Center came to an end, and frankly, from my perspective, it didn't end too soon. Master Lee was kind and compassionate, and Katherine got some good tips from him on how to continue the acupuncture treatments at home. She also had productive and validating consultations with Master Lee's son who was helpful in fine-tuning my supplement regimen. All in all it was a good visit, a productive one, but I wanted to be home—yesterday.

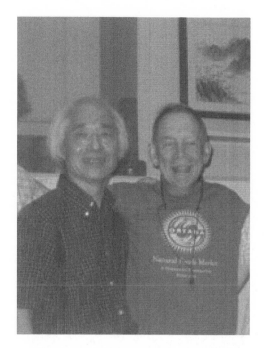

Master Lee and Greg (sans bagel!), 9/4/04.

23.

LEAP OF FAITH

KATHERINE

WHEN WE ARRIVED HOME, I left our bags in the doorway and tiptoed through the quiet house, up the short flight of stairs to my study. I remembered how we had birthed it into reality. It wasn't that long ago that it didn't exist. Real estate offerings were slim and depressing—either too much money or too many problems. Greg phoned one morning and announced he had found a house for us. I was discouraged by our futile searches and was thrilled to hear more.

"Well," he said, "it has a very open floor plan." Intrigued, I put down what I was doing to listen. "It's surrounded by yellow police tape," he went on. "The house has been in a fire, but it's on a lake." He chuckled at his humor. Great. The fire had occurred in July and the volunteer firemen had taken a half hour to get there. It really was just a burned-out shell of its former self.

"It's got a great garage and driveway!" Greg added optimistically.

I swallowed hard and agreed to come over and take a look. The decimated structure had sat open all summer, and it was a rainy October day. Those were the days when Greg was the forever optimist and I was the pessimist, needing to be convinced. Well, the rest is history. We eventually bought the place, believing that we could recycle much of what remained.

In an odd way, it was the perfect project/headache for us. We had just returned from a week at the Omega Center with spiritual teacher Thich Nhat Hahn. During the retreat, he spoke to us about the nature of impermanence, and how everything was on its way to becoming something else. He invited us to see the flower in the compost. So we un-built the house, brick by brick, and stirred the ashes, envisioning our phoenix rising. I kept imagining a room for meditation, convinced that every home needed such a room, or even just a corner, for peace. And so a meditation space wiggled its way into the design at the last moment and sat perched on top of the house—a single room banked by windows on all sides. The room was my place to learn, to write, to listen. The only problem was that there were periods of time when I didn't go there enough. Weeks would pass by. Then a long stretch would arrive and I was up there every morning, connecting to the universe, listening.

As I entered the meditation room that morning, the prayer flags hung motionless. Brenin had given them to me when he returned from Nepal, a series of brightly colored pieces of cloth, each the size of a single sheet of writing paper. They were connected in a row by a single black thread, and each one held a sacred prayer written in Nepalese. Although I couldn't read them, I knew they held wishes of peace for all beings. The people of Nepal believed that when the wind blew the flags, it cast the prayers of peace out into the universe. Tattered and weather-beaten flags reflected that much goodness had been broadcast into the world. My flags were still brightly colored and crisp.

That morning a strong wind blew across the lake, and I twisted the cranks at the base of all the windows to open them. As the cool wind rushed in, the flags fluttered and snapped. A feeling of joy filled the room, touching the flags and me. It dawned on me that things could not happen until all the conditions were just so: correct and possible. A perfect recipe existed for everything. Some ingredients came from what I decided or envisioned, and others came from some force outside me. It must be God. I had hung the prayer flags, but nothing happened until the wind was there to find them. Today my prayers were released into the wind.

I could still hear Master Lee shouting at Greg, "You not dying!" He was right—Greg was not dying. At least not now, and wasn't that all we really knew anyway? That day I held onto a glimpse of the big picture. It was the same feeling I had looking up at the night sky on a cloudless, moonless night, seeing stars within stars and glimpsing the clustering of the Milky Way. I prayed for everyone; that we might have a greater understanding of love and intimately know our highest self and feel God in the wind.

That morning I was ready and eager to do the work only I could do. I sat down at my desk and uncapped my pen. I wrote a letter to my patients to explain the direction I was heading in my life. I invited them to come along on the path that was opening before me. The words flowed onto the blank page.

The days that followed were filled with a new clarity and hard-won courage. All the questions that had been rattling around in my head, taunting and inspiring me, were finally being answered. I thought about Rilke's advice to love the questions until one day, without your noticing, they would find their way to answers. I understood how difficult it was to walk that path—like the lotus flower that began life in the dark, in the muck of the pond. Inch by inch it moved in the direction of light until one day, it opened in the still light of morning.

Three days later I met Bernie and bought the Front Street office building. It was early morning and the title company had just opened. Since our lawyer had reviewed the land contract ahead of time, we were familiar with the terms and details. We exchanged pleasantries, then tackled the forms.

I looked at Bernie and thought about the talks we'd had over the summer. He was like an old loaf of bread, crusty on the outside, kind and safe on the inside. He had shared some of his heartaches with me. His wife of thirty years had suffered a stroke one day while he was gone. He found her on the floor of their ranch house, unable to speak. She would never speak again, and died just a few days later. He told me about his son with disabilities. He didn't look at me as he explained how he had made the decision to place him in a long-term care facility.

Bernie had lived through the rough spots of life and found a way to keep going. He knew about Greg—I mean he really knew. He just nodded when I tried to explain why I was taking so long to make up my mind about the office. He never threatened to put the building on the market, opening it up to other prospective buyers. He waited for me.

He was different that day at the title company. He was squeaky clean, brusque, and in no mood for small or soft talk. For that matter, I wasn't either. I sat with my doubts and my fears, my thoughts of death and impermanence. But I led with courage. I had found a way to ride with it all in my heart and to reach out and grab the gold ring. It was my destiny, and I had to fulfill it.

The next morning I returned to my office and sat down with my soon to be ex-partner Sharon to sign legal papers. I agreed to continue to work through the coming fall as a contract employee. I gave her the Cliffs Notes version of my plans, and explained that I was creating my own office and would let my patients know as soon as I had a new phone number. There was a respectful silence between us. I didn't try to read her face for approval or permission. I didn't need it.

Emerson had her own breakthroughs. We went to her pediatrician for a well child checkup. At age three and a half, her biggest concern focused on her favorite habit—sucking her thumb. Greg was forever encouraging her to stop, telling her how hard it was on her teeth. She turned a deaf ear to our cajoling, predictions, and bribes. She was in no way ready to give it up, but she knew we were going to talk to her doctor about it.

After a perfectly normal physical exam, she hopped off the exam table and cuddled up in my lap. Dr. Olson gave her a high five and congratulated her on moving up to the next level at the Montessori Children's House. He then proclaimed that she could suck her thumb for a little while longer without any dire consequences. As I buckled her into her car seat, she said, "Let's call Daddy and tell him the happy news!" I looked into her shining eyes, sensitive to her will, and kissed her chubby thumb.

Greg took vicarious pleasure, or so it seemed, in the life surging around him. He was still unusually thin, but his appetite was picking up a bit, and he was sleeping and breathing better. He agreed to resume the arduous supplement regimen, along with regular acupuncture and laser treatments. We had brought home a small suitcase filled with individual Baggies of the medicinal tea made by Mark and Master Lee. Greg winced each time he drank their dark bitterness. The younger Dr. Lee had encouraged Greg to add a pharmaceutical grade mushroom extract that was imported from Japan. He believed it would strengthen Greg's immune system.

THERE GREW A WELCOME PEACE between Greg and myself. It was a calmness that we hadn't known for months. We knew we had done everything we could, and now it was time to wait. We relaxed into the glory of autumn.

My weeks fell into a routine of one day at the hospital, two days in the office, and now two days creating my new practice and remodeling a building. The Victorian house was perfect in many ways, but bringing it up to code and improving aesthetics were daunting projects. The asphalt siding needed to be replaced, as well as the fifteen-year-old roof. I decided to replace the simple three-step cement block entry with a covered wooden porch. The electrical system required extensive upgrading to the standards of an operating room. Microscopes, exam tables, and office furniture—the list was endless.

As part of my hospital work directing the Integrative Medicine Program, I'd arranged for Christine Page to present a community workshop on "The Courage to Change." In addition to being a medical intuitive, she was a fantastic teacher, had written several books, and lectured all over the world. She was wise and funny. At lunch I confided to her that I wanted to become more grateful. Didn't Meister Eckhart, the German theologian, say that the only prayer you ever needed to say was "thank you"? She nodded her head, lifted her glass of lemon water, and took a deep drink.

"Be careful that beneath that wish there isn't a feeling of being unworthy or undeserving," she responded. Her arrow hit the bull's eye—how did she know? Then she smiled and said, "How about instead of more gratitude, you increase celebration in your life? Like the rose in the garden, the one full of herself and her glory. Be that rose."

Later that night, as I reviewed the events of the day with Greg, he said, "Why don't we have a party at the new office?"

"What?" I asked. "The new office is just an empty building."

I knew he was right, but I still had my brakes on. How could we celebrate when we didn't know what would happen? Hadn't he been given a death sentence just five months ago?

Then I thought about Christine's counsel to me. Wasn't celebration really just a more active form of gratitude?

There was one thing I knew for sure; I was grateful for Greg sitting there with me at the dining room table.

Our lives were a long way from perfect, and our future was anything but guaranteed, but I lifted my foot from the brake and began planning the party. I gathered flowers from my garden, set up a card table with the office blueprints on it, and bought a few bottles of champagne. We invited the people who had helped us make it this far down the road, plus friends who supported us from the sidelines and our new neighbors. The gathering was perfect, and I smiled till my face hurt. Maybe I wasn't the ideal rose in the garden of life, but I felt like a glorious sunflower nodding to the sun.

GREG

FALL HAS ALWAYS BEEN MY FAVORITE TIME OF YEAR. Many people are in love with summer, an odd few even stand in favor of winter. For me, winter and summer are just too obvious; they remain so stubbornly fixed in their unchangeable and boringly predictable weather. Give me spring and fall instead, each so mutable, each full of promise of things to come. Some believe that the robins and crocuses of spring are evidence of resurrected life, while fall is the harbinger of death. But September was always the start of my new year, when summer ended and the school year began.

The fall of 2004 was a different story. Cancer had already taken so much from our lives, and that September it robbed me of my usual autumn adrenalin rush. There were still things to look forward to—football, drizzly nights with witches and goblins, the deep blush of the deciduous trees as they stripped themselves bare and tucked themselves in for the winter—but I couldn't help wondering if instead of a beginning, it would be the end.

Soon I would know, one way or the other.

I made an appointment with Dr. Nelson, my new ear, nose, and throat (ENT) doctor. (The doctor who had originally diagnosed my cancer had died after losing his own battle with cancer.) Dr. Nelson's office was located in the basement of an unappealing office building in town. There was a small waiting area, sparsely decorated with six chairs and an end table that would be difficult to sell at a yard sale.

There was a narrow hallway down the center of the suite that led to a series of compact exam rooms.

Dr. Nelson's receptionist led me into one of the exam rooms, and informed me that the doctor would be with me shortly. It was clear the building had been built before the government decreed patients have a right to privacy. I could hear every word spoken by an older couple in the room next to me. The woman was giving her husband last-minute instructions on what he should tell the doctor. The man responded to his wife's directives with a series of brief snorts, like a horse trying to spit the bit out of its mouth. Their "discussion" was cut short by a loud knock on the door.

Dr. Nelson was as modest and unassuming as his office surroundings. A rotund man of medium stature, he dressed in a frumpy white lab coat that may have been the same one he'd bought decades ago as a resident. A pencil-thin mustache bisected his full face, and on the top of his head was a thick white strap attached to a large silver mirror. He had a brusque manner, and his speech was peppered with pithy comments as he looked through my bulky chart. Dr. Nelson appeared to be his own man, not afraid to speak his mind even if it meant questioning the recommendations of the oncologists at the Cancer Center.

He might have been old school, but he was as bright as any newbie. Even though he never said so, I felt from the start that he cared about me and was invested in how I was doing. I heard a rumor that he had been diagnosed with multiple myeloma, also a devastating cancer, but he never discussed his personal struggles with me.

Dr. Nelson wasted no time completing his exam and writing an order for the PET scan and MRI of my head and neck. He didn't wish me good luck when I left his office; I got the feeling he wasn't the type of person who believed in such a thing.

THE REST OF SEPTEMBER was spent helping Emerson and Katherine transition into their new lives. Emerson was excited about moving up to a new grade level. She wanted to bring her kitty cat calculator to school; I let her take it, even though I was sure that three-year-old children didn't use calculators at school.

I thought about my mother as I watched Emerson carefully pack her red backpack. My mother had been so sick for so long—as far back as I could remember. When all four of her children finally crossed the line into adulthood, she confessed that she had achieved her goal, which was to live long enough to see all of us graduate from high school.

My mother and I differed from each other, and we followed our own paths to be sure. Yet we'd somehow found ourselves in the same place, teetering on the edge between life and death, both wishing we could live long enough to see our children graduate. She made it, and now it was my turn. If only I could live for fourteen more years! I imagined myself watching with pride as Emerson climbed up on the stage to claim her diploma!

Living fourteen years felt impossible, like counting to infinity.

Katherine held fast to her dream of buying a building for her new practice, however, and that fall I watched with pride as she brought it to reality. We discussed her laundry list of worries: *Can I make it? Will people come and see me?* I had absolutely no doubt about her chances for success. In fact, my fear was just the opposite. I was afraid she would be deluged with work. People were hungry for her kind of medicine, the true healing kind that comes from the heart rather than the ego.

On September 9, Katherine signed the dotted line and purchased the building. We grabbed the keys, drove over to the property. There are certain people, such as architects and designers, who can visualize how different living rooms or kitchens would look. Katherine's gift was different; she was born with a sixth sense. She could feel when things were right, what they were "meant to be." She would talk about a magnetic-like resonance toward certain people and situations, and describe how she felt pulled in this way or that. I learned early on to trust her intuition. After all, it was her intuition that brought us together in the first place, and led us to conceive Emerson on that auspicious night on Maui.

I watched through a filter of moist eyes as Katherine climbed the steps of the old Victorian house and paused in the doorway. She knew she had found the right place, and I knew it too.

24.
SOUL'S DECISION

KATHERINE

DAWN BECKONED ME from my desk to the outside world. I walked onto the dock just as the sun broke through the cloud bank, transforming the sky into a majestic palate of colors: fiery reds, burnt corals, and bruised purples. The lake was losing the last of its heat, and a fine mist condensed just above its surface in the brisk morning air. My bare feet felt every drop of the cold dew, and I wrapped my robe tighter. I stood motionless at the end of the dock and witnessed God all around me. Turning to look back at the house, I saw Greg standing in the doorway. His arm rose in a wave, and then he patted his heart with a gentle motion of his hand. Our love was the prayer flag that we waved at each other that morning. Not only had it survived, it had grown stronger.

The days fluttered by like the amber leaves dropping from the trees. The roadside markets offered up pumpkins, bushels of apples, and shocks of corn stalks. Emerson and I went for a horse-drawn carriage ride through the old hospital grounds that remained in the center of town. The surrounding forests and hillsides were at their autumn finest.

I flowed through the agendas that sprouted up day and night. Greg was still unable to sleep, and I continued to give him treatments in the night. He preferred the laser, as the needles felt too harsh in the darkness. Just as he was falling asleep, Emerson would call out and plead for me to lie beside her for just a moment or two.

All the hopping from bed to bed didn't stop my dreams. They only became more vivid and penetrating. There was one dream that stood out:

Greg and I were staying in a one-room house in Africa with a family. They were native bush people, and the father, a no-nonsense kind of guy, captivated me. He lived with awareness and restraint. As I looked into our bags filled with insignificant odds and ends, I decided not to unpack them, certain they would only clutter their small home. Greg sat with the father and shared the details of a presentation he was working on, the culmination of his life's work. The man encouraged Greg to think bigger. Then, without warning, we needed to leave to make a connection. The father was now more impish in nature, and paid for my fare with someone else's tokens.

I woke up. What did the dream mean? It felt like spirit travel. Certainly, it introduced a new authority figure to my journey.

I decided it was asking me to simplify, and to be careful with what I unpacked. The old man reminded me that I was mining an inner discipline; one that inspired awareness in others, an inner reflection, a longing for a deeper knowing. Yet he was also a playful presence, looking into your face, curious who you were and what made your eyes sparkle. It was not exactly a business plan, but that's what it felt like to me.

In mid-October we contemplated Greg going back to work with Master Lee, who was leaving for Korea. It would be months before he returned to Boston. We couldn't figure out the flights or the logistics, and in the end, Greg chose to stay home. Jim came for a weekend, and they spent their time watching college football, eating Greg's famous electric chili, and walking around the peninsula at its peak of color. Greg laughed and played and took us on boat rides around the lake at sunset. It was his way of healing.

October 26th approached, the day Greg was scheduled to have his PET scan. It was a heart-wrenching time, and we considered not going through with the test. We wrestled with the agony of knowing and the anxiety of not knowing. We could not decide which was worse. Had the cancer slowed down? How many days did he have left? Finally, I convinced us both that we needed to know the truth, one way or the other. I looked into Greg's blue eyes and said, "You want to know, don't you? Otherwise you will always be thinking the worst. You have already faced the most difficult outcome in your thoughts. We need to know."

Greg knew it was the right decision but he was afraid. He dressed quickly in the dark bedroom and drove to the radiology clinic alone. He wanted to do it that way, and, I guess, maybe it was best for me too.

GREG

THE INFUSION CLINIC WAS BUSTLING the morning I went for my PET scan. Both the PET scan and MRI required that I have an IV placed in my arm. I scheduled the scans a scant 24 hours apart with the hope that I would only have to get jabbed once. I could have gone directly to the PET scan clinic and had the stupid IV put in there, but instead I chose to go to the infusion clinic, assuming that the nurses there had more experience with needles.

A chill came over me as I sat in the waiting room, and I noticed that the noises behind the receptionist window seemed to be getting louder. My heart was racing and my armpits moistened. The clinic's interior door opened to reveal a nurse holding a chart. She seemed to shout out my name. "Gregory Holmes?" I raised my hand like a nervous child in a classroom. The nurse smiled broadly and encouraged me to follow her.

We walked by several patients sitting in recliners, receiving their doses of chemotherapy. The nurse had me sit in a recliner too, and listened as I recounted for the umpteenth time my fear of needles. She fetched two light cotton blankets, wrapped them around my petrified body, and placed a warm compress over the target area on my left arm.

I needed to shift my focus from the impending disaster, so I asked her about herself. Like most people, she accepted the invitation and proudly chatted about her children and her husband who owned a body shop. She never forgot the visit's purpose, however, and as she told her stories she prepared the needle site.

"Ready?" she asked. I nodded, but started to weep. I couldn't help it. The needle hurt, of course, but that wasn't all I was crying about. So many tributaries fed my river of grief that day. Katherine and I had fought so hard, and we had lost so much.

The PET scan clinic was located on a separate medical campus across town. The tech was surprised when I checked in with an IV already dangling from my arm. I explained my one-poke strategy to him, and my plans for the MRI the next day. I walked up the ramp into the machine like a pirate walking the plank.

I gingerly unclasped the Saint Peregrine medal that I had not removed since David had given it to me. The tech injected a radioactive glucose liquid, the bait for the cancer cells to feed on and identify themselves. He retreated to the control booth with its thick-walled protection.

I thought about Mary and the blue balloon, and how both of them floated high above me at the Cancer Center. Mary had been so kind, and I hoped she was okay with all the radiation buzzing around her.

I scanned the technician's face as he unstrapped me from the exam table, anxiously looking for any sign of what he may or may not have seen. After all, the techs weren't stupid; they must see something on their computer monitors. But his poker face deflected my probing, and he maintained his noncommittal stance as he helped me re-clasp the medal around my neck. I walked into the men's dressing room, threw my gown into the laundry bin, and sat down in my skivvies on the cold metallic bench. I grabbed the silver medallion, held it firmly against my left cheek, and pleaded for a miracle.

Sliding the IV under the long sleeve of my dress shirt, I cinched my belt on my pants up to the very last notch, and headed off to work. Now it became my turn to maintain a neutral façade while listening to my patients' woes. I don't know how I managed to sit still that day, but I did.

KATHERINE

I THOUGHT OF DAYS PAST FROM MY RESIDENCY when I stood at the bedside of someone on the edge of death. I would be called there by my beeper or the overhead speaker, and enter the room breathing hard from the run or the flight up the stairs taken two at a time. A mixture of dread and purpose filled me. Our attempts to resuscitate life with oxygen, compressions, and IV fluids would begin immediately as the crash cart was summoned. Each person's role was determined by either who got there first or the amount of experience they had. I had done it all, from being in command and calling out directives to standing in the shadows.

Almost always a part of me rose above the commotion and drifted surreally about the room. I would send a message, a prayer, to the person's soul, "I will keep your body open while you decide. Is it time to leave? Or do you need to stay?" Then I waited and watched our human efforts until some greater decision was made. I felt like that now in a very personal way. It was up to Greg's soul. We had done everything we could.

I picked Emerson up early from school and we went shopping at our local food co-op. I was looking at the broccoli, trying to decide which head to pick up, when my pager went off. I absent-mindedly pulled the small black contraption off my belt and read the text message: "PET scan normal," followed by the name of the radiologist, "Dr. Cover: Ext 5234."

All the air went out of me. Normal? Normal! Oh my God, can this be true? No metastasis? No spread of the cancer? I looked at Emerson sitting in front of me in the cart and tickled her gently. "It's normal!" I squealed. She smiled at me, and the broccoli in her hand suddenly turned into a bouquet of flowers.

By the time we drove home, I was floating around the kitchen, unpacking the groceries in a state of disbelief and euphoria. Then I thought about it more carefully. The message "PET scan normal," meant that the cancer hadn't spread to distant sites—but what about his sinus area where the tumor was in the first place? What did that show? I put Emerson down for her nap and nervously dialed Dr. Cover's extension.

I heard his voice. "Hello Dr. Cover! It's Katherine. I wanted to go over Greg's scan with you if that's okay? I don't think it's a HIPPA violation as he definitely has given me permission to discuss it with you."

"No problem," he said. "I saw the study come through the department and took the pleasure of reading it. There was no uptake on the scan."

I stared into space and repeated, "No uptake? Anywhere? Not even in the previous areas? I mean, the sinus area?" I waited, holding my breath.

"Yep, even the sinus area is clear!" His voice was kind and sincere. "Best news I've given anyone all day. I'm so happy for both of you. Let me know if I can help you in any way!"

From the bottom of my heart, and in the spirit of Meister Eckhart, my mouth found the words, "Thank you!"

All the walls that I had built to brace myself for possible outcomes crumbled. My face melted into my hands and I burst into tears. I thought of Emerson's words, "Let's call Daddy and tell him the happy news." I choked as I did. That night Greg and I held each other and sobbed. Emerson stood beside us, looking frightened by our naked display of emotion. With tear-streaked faces, we reassured her that they were happy tears. No moment had ever been more sweet or more laced with tragedy.

GREG

I FELT A SENSE OF EXTREME URGENCY in Katherine's message on my answering machine. "Greg!" she exclaimed. "Call me!" I could tell something was wrong, and I knew what that something was. She had gotten word of my PET scan results, and it had to be bad; after all, if it were good news she would have said so in her message.

I stood there for several minutes and glared at the small black box like it was an evil messenger. I didn't want to hear the news, but she wanted me to call her, so I gave in and punched our home number into the phone pad.

She answered the phone. "Hi honey," I said in a small, tentative voice.

"Are you sitting down?' she queried.

SHIT! I knew it! The whole thing was coming to an end just as it had begun ….

Katherine stopped that train of thought before it left the depot. "I just got off the phone with Dr. Cover," she continued, her voice climbing, full of energy. "He read the results of your PET scan! Greg, it's normal!"

"Normal?" For a moment I didn't understand what she was saying.

"Greg, it's normal," she repeated. "Dr. Cover read your scan, and couldn't find any cancer. Greg, it's gone!"

I couldn't talk. The room started to spin. I could hear Katherine's voice calling to me from a distance. "Greg…Greg. . . Greg! Are you there?"

I didn't know where I was, but I knew where I wanted to be. I told her I was coming home right away and hung up the phone. I can't tell you how I got home that day; all I can say is that Flow must have known the way.

I walked through the front door and ran into Katherine's embrace. We did it! We'd fought so hard! We started sobbing and our bodies shook as we hugged.

That night I asked Katherine to repeat everything that Dr. Cover had said. I clung to her every word like a drowning man hanging onto a life preserver. I wanted to believe that what he said was true, that the cancer was gone, but was it really? I was afraid that the all-knowing MRI would find the tumor, and I just couldn't handle the rug being pulled out from under me.

I tossed and turned that night as I went back and forth through an unending list of what ifs: What if they had mixed my PET scan up with someone else's? What if the radiologist had made a mistake? What if the MRI tomorrow found the cancer?

There was a "what if" too difficult to imagine, one that was beyond belief. What if I wasn't sick anymore? What if Katherine and I had won the fight?

The next day came not a moment too soon. The MRI tech strapped me in. He left the room, closed the lead door, and reappeared in the control booth. His disembodied voice interrupted the public radio talk show on my headphones. "Are you ready?" he asked.

Ready? I was ready all right. Ready to be done with everything: cancer, doctors, nightmares…everything! I gave him a thumb's up, and the table slid into the belly of the beast. The machine began to rumble and there were several intervals of loud beeps. After 45 minutes or so, the table rolled out of the machine and the tech came and removed the IV, setting me free. I looked deeply into his eyes for an answer, but he kept the same practiced poker face as the PET scan tech before him. He wished me well as I left for the dressing room.

I went home, where Katherine and I waited hour after hour for the test results…and then we waited some more. The neuro-radiologist needed to review the MRI along with the PET scan, and compare them to the previous images. I paced the floor, waiting for his call.

Finally, it came. The radiologist carefully explained that the previous area of solid tumor now appeared to be a fluid like substance. The places that had shown extension into my skull were no longer evident. He concluded with the verdict: "There had been a remarkable change." There was no evidence of cancer—not in my sinus cavity, my brain, or anywhere.

The bizarre premonition that came to me that dark night in the cottage turned out to be true after all! Like Ali, Katherine and I had won the fight! The tumor departed just as it arrived, offering neither explanation nor apology.

I was so excited! I wanted to shout out the good news to the world! I was going to live after all!

Suddenly the recurring nightmare that had dogged me for the past year made perfect sense. I was stunned as the puzzle pieces fell into place. How could I have missed it? I was the disabled jet that was falling out of the sky. I made the miraculous landing. I survived. Now I was eager to find a phone and tell everyone I was okay, just like in the dream.

Weird! I wondered if the nightmare had been an unconscious wish, as Freud would argue, or if someone or something were trying to tell me everything would be okay? And what was the deal, anyway, with the epiphany at Silver Lake and my strange connection with Ali?

I picked up the phone. I didn't have all the answers that night, but there were a couple of things I knew for sure. Like Ali, I had roared back from certain defeat and had given the cancer a good whupping. Ali had a great trainer in Angelo Dundee; I had Katherine in my corner. My dad was right: it had been a good fight.

KATHERINE

WHEN I HEARD THE ALL CLEAR from the radiologist, I knew a miracle had occurred. A miracle! Something opened and something else collapsed inside of me. I could and I couldn't understand it. I felt weakened by all we had undergone, yet strengthened. I believed in miracles, and had deeply prayed for one, but never before had the miraculous touched me so clearly. It was closer than a front row seat. It had occurred directly through us and to us.

For days after we received the test results, I was overcome with exhaustion and an odd irritability. Even as a young child I was at my best in the midst of a crisis, and I would collapse in the aftermath. I had thrown myself in front of Greg's cancer and given it everything I had, and even more than I knew I had. Besides all the effort, there had been another force, one that flowed through me and the many variables of the last six months. There was a presence that showed up when we were wise enough to welcome it. I thought of Andy Martin, of Muhammad Ali, of the doctors and the nurses, of Libby and Master Lee. I nodded to all the knowledge and the skill that I had witnessed and been given.

Now we were being given some time. A new truth slowly softened around me. No longer did I need to separate from the man I loved, and Emerson did not have to say goodbye to her daddy. But in this reality there was new knowledge. There would be a day, another day, when our bodies would perish. The blissful innocence that we existed forever in this form was gone, replaced by a larger, more mysterious truth. Yet, the sweet perfections of this life were all I needed now.

A good friend said, "You have been given some breathing room." I let out the breath that I had been holding in the pit of my stomach for months and smiled. Much had been taken, yet so much remained.

PART THREE

"Though much is taken, much abides;

and though

We are not now that strength which in old days

Moved earth and heaven;

that which we are, we are;

One equal temper of heroic hearts,

Made weak by time and fate, but strong in will

To strive, to seek, to find, and not to yield."

—Alfred Tennyson

25.
A CLEARING IN THE WOODS

KATHERINE

YES, WE WERE GIVEN SOME BREATHING ROOM, and I had much to contemplate. Something we did had made a difference, but what was it? What worked? How could we know? Greg and I talked many times about the complexity of his program. We ultimately agreed that there was nothing we felt ready to stop, so we kept on with renewed intensity.

What had I learned living through his diagnosis, our fight, and the resurrection? I remembered the dark April night, standing in the kitchen, holding his face in my hands and asking, "Why do we have to do this?"

The question was important to me and now I had a glimpse of the answer. My quest for healing was interwoven with Greg's. We were twin serpents on the Rod of Asclepius, the symbol from antiquity still used today in medicine and healing. The ancient symbol of the snake entwined with the staff spoke of the inseparableness of death and life. But what had it meant? My dream on December 15th, 2004 gave me a glimpse of the answer.

Emerson and I were standing on the balcony of an apartment house looking out across the water. There was a ship in the distance and Greg was on it. Somehow the boat crashed into the building on the opposite shore. All the houses tumbled with an impact creating a tsunami-like tremor, which moved in a wave across the expanse of water and slammed into our shore. I ran to brace myself with Emerson in

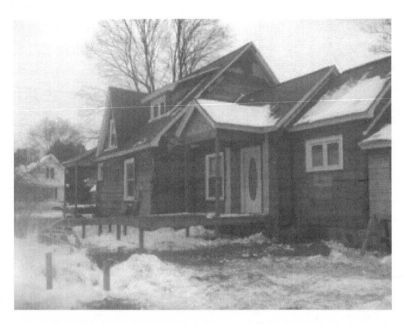

Katherine's Front Street practice under construction, Winter 2004.

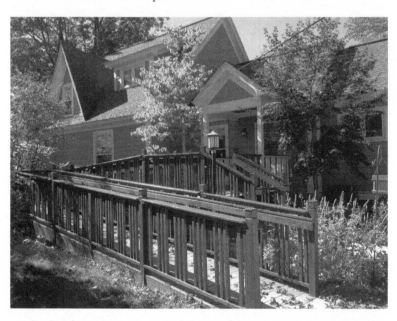

Katherine's office, 2013.

*my arms. I knew that we had survived but I couldn't see the boat. I
was frantic as I ran to get help, but no one would help me. The other
people locked their doors and ignored my pounding and shouts. I only
wanted to know whether Greg was all right.*

I woke with the dread of unknowing.

Greg's illness had sent a tidal wave of awakening in me. It was intertwined with the destruction of my own reality, like the collapsing
building. My people had locked their doors and my pleas for help
were met with resistance. I was alone with my daughter in my arms.
All I knew that December was that my previous reality crumbled.
I couldn't see what had been destroyed, or what was left standing. I
didn't know what remained. It was out of the ruble that I was found.

What found me? Teachers, friends, my son, poetry, and sunrises
unquestionably sustained me. But at the end of the day I faced the
fact that my path must be walked alone. There was no one there
for me to lean on, defer to or hide behind. As I fell into that truth,
the universe reverberated back to me. Torches flickered in the forest
along the dimly lit trail. I followed them.

Why we had to do this meant different things for each of us. For
me, it meant believing in myself to the exclusion of—maybe even
despite of—the outside world. I knew I was different from other
doctors thirty years ago when I entered the medical profession. I
wanted the knowledge and the creditability that learning medicine
would provide, yet I also wanted to be a healer. I wanted to go to the
source of illness and nurture the antidote, the wellness. I knew all
this then and I still know this.

Maybe you could call it my sixth sense. It was hard to identify
at first because it wasn't one of the five that I was familiar with. It
wasn't a voice, color, or a smell, it was a sense of resonance—a bodi-
ly sensation, a feeling of rightness and of belonging. I hadn't completely trusted my sixth sense until now. With Greg's illness, it was

all I had. At the end of day, I was forced to walk alone, and I finally and deeply trusted the path I choose.

GREG BECAME MORE INVOLVED with the supplements, and learned the names of many of them. Previously, I'd gotten up each morning to arrange the day's pills on the kitchen counter, but now he helped me organize them. We dumped a month's worth of supplements onto the basement floor, and as we worked, the carpet became covered with hundreds of small piles of colorful pills: orange, green, amber, brown, and white. We sorted them according to the time of day he needed to take them, then put them into empty bottles. Greg called it a "medicine factory," and it really did feel like it.

One afternoon I noticed that Greg's hands looked yellow. Was he jaundiced from an injured liver? When I looked more carefully, I realized that the yellow stain on his skin had come from handling the curcumin pills. I laughed. I loved that I could laugh again.

That fall I became absorbed and enthralled with creating my new office. Over the months, I'd made thousands of decisions: I picked out the paint colors, the mirrors, the exam tables, the baby scales, the centrifuge, the art, the doorknobs—the list was endless. But each decision was like a brush stroke, helping to bring my vision more clearly into focus. Without advertising, I found and hired two wonderful women to assist me in the running of the office. With the help of my friend, Angela, a graphic artist, I created my logo. The symbol is a variation of an ancient one that means "welcome" and "blessing for a long life."

Even though I would be practicing family medicine in an outpatient setting, there were building codes for everything—electrical wiring, exit lighting, handicap ramps, and water fountains. I refused to become discouraged by the endless and inflexible rules, although I did break into tears once with frustration. Instead, I focused on the intention, the vision, and the love.

The last week of February 2005 brought us the culmination of a lifetime. Greg had a repeat MRI, and it showed no sign of cancer. The radiologist now referred to "post surgical changes" in the previous area of cancer. A few days later I opened the doors of my new office and began to see my first patients with a joy I did not know was possible. After all the hard work, the sleepless nights, and the slow careful attention to envisioning every detail in my head, the reality of actually walking into it was like entering a dream. I will never forget the magic and the mystery of it.

My work continues, and new patients continue to seek me out. I work daily to bridle the busyness of my life. I fight to not take it for granted. I remember most of the time to run to greet Greg on ordinary days. This is the story I promised to share, and I am honored to tell. If it helps one person, my efforts will not have been in vain.

GREG

I WOULD LOVE TO TELL YOU that our story ended like this: That after six grueling months of fighting our war with cancer, we won! That the ravenous cancer cells, once strong and arrogant, were now dead, gone for good, and that Katherine and I, victorious, drove off into a rose-colored sunset and lived happily ever after. But that isn't what happened. The truth of the matter is that there is no Hollywood ending to our story, no grand finale where our friends and family came together to celebrate and sing songs of joy.

Here's what really happened. Although Katherine and I were shocked and overjoyed by the unbelievable news that October, we were also aware that in many ways our fight was far from over. We could not afford to let our guard down and assume that the cancer was gone forever. The grim reality was that the odds remained firmly stacked in the cancer's favor, and that rogue cancer cells were in the process of regrouping and planning another attack.

Our war with cancer hasn't really ended. Wars linger in the deep recesses of memory long after the cease-fire, ready to be reignited at a moment's notice by any small trigger. During my internship on the post-traumatic stress unit I witnessed soldiers return from the rice paddies of Vietnam, only to bring the war home with them. These were the forgotten soldiers, the uncounted casualties. Loss and grief were the order of the day: Some of the soldiers lost their limbs, many of them their buddies, and most of them their faith. Every one of them believed they were losing their minds. Any sense of innocence or naïveté that the soldiers may have had before going overseas was destroyed, replaced by an explosive combination of cynicism, hostility, and mistrust. Small, everyday events—small to you and me—immediately sent the soldiers hurtling back into harm's way. The sharp crack of a car backfire was the telltale sound of an assassin's rifle, the booming Fourth of July fireworks a sure sign of incoming shells.

One of the biggest casualties I suffered during my war was a loss of confidence in my health. Gone were the worry-free healthy days before cancer. Now, I lived in a state of constant fear of another attack. The cancer had raped me; it had entered my body against my will, robbed me of my health, and destroyed my trust in my body's ability to ward off future attackers. The freedom from disease that I never fully appreciated was replaced by an unrelenting hyper-vigilance. Every little ache and pain that I'd once thought of as no more than an inconvenience was now a sure sign of cancer.

I was the one who had become a frightened war veteran. I scanned my face several times a day in the bathroom mirror, carefully comparing each side, convinced more often than not that the left side of my face was bigger, swollen, different in some telltale, pathologic way. Katherine would need to remind me of Master Lee's prescient words, "You not dying!"

My post-war problems didn't end there. I suffered serious collateral damage from the friendly fire of the chemo and radiation. My thyroid gland was completely decimated, and that meant adding yet another pill to my already enormous pile of daily supplements. The hearing in my left ear was about half of what it had been before I was nuked by the radiation, and my sense of smell was almost gone. I developed dry eye syndrome in my left eye, making it vulnerable to chronic infections.

We sent copies of the PET scan and MRI to Dr. Abdul at the Cancer Center for his blessing. He emailed back within a week or so. His conclusion after reading them was far less sanguine. He was unmoved by the dramatic absence of the tumor from my sinus cavity. Instead he commented on a small area at the base of my skull that appeared abnormal. Dr. Abdul failed to say whether he thought it was cancer, and he recommended that I have an MRI of my head and neck every six months for the indefinite future.

This was not the "all clear" that I needed to hear. In fact, it was just the opposite, and it poured fuel on the fire of my worry. I shared my concerns with my local ENT, Dr. Nelson. He called the radiology department at the local hospital and spoke directly with the neuro-radiologist who had dictated my report. The radiologist did not share Dr. Abdul's opinion, and said that it was normal for people to have that particular finding on their scan.

I regretted sending my scans to Dr. Abdul. Not only had I wanted him to confirm that the cancer was gone, but I'd also wanted him to be happy for me, to gush over me like the proud parent of a child with a straight-A report card. I knew from our past interactions that expressing feelings (assuming he had them) was simply not his thing, yet I still wanted him be different, and his being different was about as likely as E.T. landing in my backyard. What in the world was I thinking? After all, didn't Einstein claim that the definition of insanity was doing the same thing again and again and expecting different results? The bottom-line is that he and I were opposites;

I needed him to be reassuring, optimistic, and caring, whereas he needed to remain cautious, certain, and withholding.

I just wanted one oncologist to tell me that I was cured forever! End of scans, end of exams, end of discussion! But doctors shy away from using the four-letter "c" word when it comes to cancer. They prefer noncommittal phrases instead, the ones with less liability, such as "in remission" and "decreased likelihood of reoccurrence." Personally, I hated the phrase "in remission" because it meant temporary recovery, an intermission if you will, and there was no way in hell that I wanted to see the second part of the show.

As for "temporary," I didn't want my recovery to be temporary; I wanted it to last forever, like most things: my marriage, being a parent to Emerson, the survival of the planet. I knew full well that nothing really lasts forever, that all things must pass, that everything has a season. But it was my season, and I vowed to do everything in my power to make it endure as long possible.

Oncologists measure cancer survival in terms of years, with intervals of three and five years being the high-water marks. When I was first diagnosed, I measured survival in much smaller increments: days, weeks, six to twelve months, max. To think that I might make it three or five years was preposterous.

Armed with the miraculous news from the scans, I began to cautiously extend my horizon and started thinking in terms of six-month increments. Katherine and I returned to our practices that fall with a renewed sense of hope and purpose. My appetite slowly returned from its hiatus. I was able to gain some much-needed weight, and even added a bit of muscle from workouts at the gym. I was still unsteady on the treadmill, but I felt more like a newborn colt trying to run on spindly legs than an old grey mare headed to the glue factory.

ONE OF THE HARDEST THINGS about being a cancer "survivor" is watching other people die. At times I had pangs of guilt that I'd survived when others didn't. The veterans at the VA talked about having "survivors guilt," a self-reproach that they had made it back alive while their buddies came home in flag-draped boxes. Some felt that they hadn't deserved to live, and at times their feelings of guilt and shame would become so intense, so unremitting, and so painful they would attempt suicide. Or bury their feelings with drugs and alcohol.

June of the next year brought the expected, yet unacceptable, death of our good friend David. He'd been very ill with cancer for quite some time, and the cancer treatments at the end only seemed to cause him and his wife Cynthia additional pain and suffering.

I remember when Cynthia informed us that David had only days to live. It was important to Katherine and me that we see him one last time and say our goodbyes to our dear friend, an exceedingly generous soul, and person who had been the poster child for living life large. We jumped in the car and headed downstate.

The bright evergreen forests of Northern Michigan gave way to farmlands, which in turn yielded to the ubiquitous concrete of metropolitan Lansing. My pulse quickened as we made our final approach into David and Cynthia's neighborhood. I felt like a little kid inside, kicking and screaming, not wanting to go, not wanting to do something I knew I had to do. I didn't want to walk through the doorway of my denial and face the cold fact that another one of my great friends was dying.

It was an ominous sign when Cynthia met us at the door instead of David. He was in the living room, tilted back in his recliner, looking off into the distance. He was still alive, but it was clear that his bag was packed for whatever came next.

"David . . ." I began gingerly, searching for the right words that don't exist. "It's Greg and Katherine . . ."

"Yes," was his short reply. I knew immediately that a big part of him—the garrulous, expansive, verbose part—was already gone. What energy remained seemed meditative, reflective, and introverted. The deafening silence that followed spoke volumes.

I sat next to him and tried to hold onto what was left. I swear I could feel life energy leaving his body. Finally he interrupted the silence and pronounced, "You know, dying is not such a bad thing—people have been doing it for centuries." I didn't know exactly what he meant, but it felt like David had come to some important conclusion after years of spiritual search.

I wanted to stay right next to him, forever. I knew it would be the last time I saw him alive. Saying goodbye to him that day was like casting off a rope on a boat that was ready to head across the seas to a foreign land. As I reached over to give him a final hug, David quietly spoke his last words to me, "Such a good man."

When Katherine and I left David's house I thought about how cancer, like a sniper, had picked off another one of my dear friends. First Marilyn, and now David. A chill came over me as I stared out the car window. I was sure I wasn't far back in line.

IT WAS JUST A FEW MONTHS AFTER DAVID DIED that I saw God. I'm not kidding you, I really did see God—at least that's what I believe. One night I had a dream that was quite unlike any dream before or since. The clarity of the dream itself was unbelievable, and the special effects were far more spectacular than any computer-generated movie imagery. It was so amazing, so compelling, and so unforgettable that I knew it was a true vision.

I was alone in a car traveling down a road in the countryside south of East Lansing in the middle of the night. I was trying my best to catch Marilyn and David, who were in a car in front of me. Suddenly their car darted off onto a dirt two-track that went through a large pasture and into a grove of trees on the top of a hill. They got out of their car and started walking along a winding trail through the dark forest until they came to a small clearing.

I followed them along the path, but for some reason I couldn't catch up to them. Then, suddenly, Marilyn and David jumped into the middle of the clearing, clasped each other's hands, and disappeared into a wild vortex of beautiful lights made up of different colors. The swirling lights were accompanied by harmonic tones that were beyond my wildest imagination. They were magnificent, intense, and overwhelming. As I watched Marilyn and David dissolve into the light, I was overcome by a powerful feeling of infinite love. It was more than I could handle, and I dropped to the ground, paralyzed by feelings I couldn't process. I began weeping. I felt as though I had been hit by some kind of spiritual Taser.

When I woke up that morning I was still weeping. I knew I had witnessed something that was beyond incredible. Marilyn had kept the promise she'd made to me that night in the hot tub after all! She came back to show me that there was life after death!

Marilyn and David had spent a great deal of their lives in a diligent search for the divine, and they had found it. After my vision that night, I was sure that I had too.

I was so relieved to find out that the afterlife was different from the one pitched to me in my childhood by the nuns. There were no pearly gates, no Saint Peter, no condo on the beach for good people. And I never did believe that God looked like some burly, buffed-up version of Santa Claus. Marilyn and David had become something much greater than anything I could ever imagine.

I lost my fear of death that night, but I've never lost my love for life. I do agree with the nuns and priests that heaven and hell exist, but I don't believe they happen after you die; I believe that they happen here, on Earth, while we are alive. I went through heaven and hell during my battle with cancer. It was hell losing two irreplaceable friends from cancer, it was hell being diagnosed with cancer and going through the treatments.

But even through all the pain, misery, and loss I still had my moments of heaven. Of course, there were the obvious times, like my epiphany at Silver Lake that I would beat the tumor, and the day when I found out that the tumor was gone. Those were indeed heavenly. Yet I'm truly grateful for my newfound ability to appreciate the not-so-obvious miracles in my daily life, such as the pair of cardinals that perch on my office window feeder every day, and the majesty of the clean lakes and forests that surround me. I feel the deepest gratitude for Katherine, and the love and support of my family and friends. It's been said that a person doesn't fully appreciate something until it's gone. I am so thankful that I have been given a second chance.

I'm not ready to go into that mystical forest clearing and be one with Marilyn and David, caught up in heaven's infinite love. All that can wait. What I really want is one more day of heaven on Earth, one more day of being Emerson's dad. One more night to snuggle with Katherine, my soul mate, my hero, the doctor who saved my life.

KATHERINE

NO DOCTOR EVER HAS ASKED GREG OR ME what we did in his battle with cancer. Not one! If they did what would I say? Which piece of our program made a difference? Looking back over the years of treatment, I realize we wove a tapestry. Each thread counted and created the mysterious powerful pattern.

There were so many threads. The easiest to identify was the physical dimension. The first physical thread was to decrease the inflammation in his body. This involved nurturing his digestion, eating a low sugar, good oil diet, plus consuming nutrients that were anti-inflammatory such as curcumin, green tea, resveratrol, astathaxin, milk thistle, and many antioxidants, especially vitamin D.

The second physical thread was increasing Greg's circulation while simultaneously decreasing stagnation. He was able to do this with regular exercise, massage and enzyme supplements that encouraged blood flow and fluidity, such as bromelain, serretia peptidase, and lumbrokinase.

The third thread was balancing his immune system into active vigilance with acupuncture and mushroom extracts. We continuously found ways to improve sleep and restoration, as well as relaxation. Medicinal Chinese herbs, such as Magnolia officialis, rehmannia, astralagus taken morning and night worked to restore yin and calm shen.

All of those threads were important. My antennae were always up as I continued to read, listen, and explore. I literally felt nudged into selecting nutrients when I listened to my sixth sense. True, it was an educated sense, but I felt drawn to read certain articles over others, or listen to particular healers. In this way, I would discover a new piece of information that wove into our plan.

There were the emotional threads. We were very fortunate in this regard. From the moment of the illness, we knew we would be there for each other. There was an unshakeable trust between us. It sobered me when I learned how marriages ended or how partners were abandoned when they were diagnosed with cancer. Illness is not for the weak of heart.

Love is often confused with infatuation and magical thinking of how the other will complete us. In reality it has so much more to do with making choices and taking action for the growth and fulfillment of the other. Over the years, I learned firsthand about the discipline of love. I learned to love in a way that did not neglect the self, but rather enlarged it by making the choice to help another.

Ralph Waldo Emerson spoke of the moral inclination that leads to the enlightened spiritual heart. My moral inclination, my higher self, watered that love and I discovered its power would show up during difficult times, even when I didn't think that I could.

Love is such a core ingredient of healing. Love in relationship with others, but, equally if not more so, love of the self. Are we worthy of love? Do we love ourselves? Love means making decisions and taking steps that support our growth and fulfillment. I was on the path of self-love by removing the barriers of guilt and lack of confidence. Greg was learning that he was worth fighting for at his very core.

Finally, there was the thread of the will and the spirit. Do you want to live? A diagnosis of cancer is the strongest litmus test I know. People must be fiercely determined to survive. I ask them this question when I meet them. They could be 32 years old or 92. I never assume that I know their answer.

There have been times when I have asked, and with relief, the patient has confessed that they don't want to go on living. They have even asked permission to not keep fighting. They have quietly admitted that they are feeling drawn to be with a sister or brother who has already passed, or that they are at peace with the fullness of their life. Some are not sure. But there are those who look me in the eye and declare unwaveringly that they want to live. I encourage them to do everything they can, but know that even then there is no guarantee.

We cannot know when it's our time to die. But I believe that if you don't try—really try—to live, the chances of surviving are much less. We must not back down from the seriousness or complexity of what is being asked of us. Occasionally patients balk, complaining that it is just too much…too many pills, too much work, or too much money. Unfortunately, I understand this, and I admit I have on occasion tried to make it easier for them. I don't tell them all that I can, or how hard it can be. They want the simplicity of one supplement or one food to save them. They fight with one hand tied behind their back and aren't ready to fight fire with fire.

But it's not that easy. They must do everything to create a body where cancer cannot thrive. Greg was the master of this commandment. He had his moments, but the overarching effort he displayed every day to live was staggering. He kept the vow he'd made to me in the Cancer Center. He would do anything and everything to live.

The world is ready for a more comprehensive approach to cancer. We must demand more care of the environment and more cautionary research with the use of chemicals, pesticides, and herbicides. Our goal must be to prevent cancer from beginning in the first place.

People are hungry for a more holistic treatment of cancer. We must respect the healers who are working to find ways to use natural substances, along with chemotherapy and radiation, to make treatment less toxic and more effective. I encourage anyone with cancer to seek out people who are passionate and knowledgeable about this growing area of research.

I RECENTLY HEARD AN INTERVIEW with poet and writer, Gary Snyder, on public radio. Gary talked about an experience he'd had when he was 25 years old and studying in Japan. He had been directed to a sect of monks who lived in the remote mountains. Their initiation rite included hanging him upside down with a rope tied around his feet. As he dangled over a mountain cliff, they asked him important life questions. The interviewer prodded further about what he was asked. Gary said quietly, "Oh, I don't think I should talk about that."

There was mirth and wisdom in his voice, and it resonated deeply within me. I believe in each of our lives there will come a time when we are hung over a cliff. It might be cancer, war, or the loss of someone or something precious that brings us there. We will be asked important questions. I can't tell you what the questions will be, and I certainly can't tell you the answers. I can tell you that you must prepare for the asking...and live your life discovering the answers.

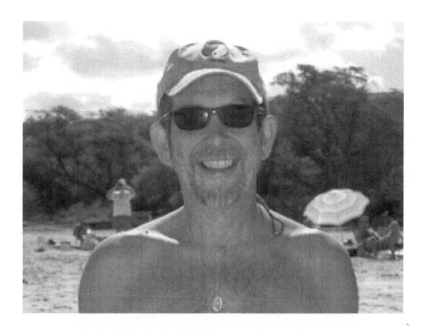

Greg in Hawaii with the Saint Peregrine medal from David, 2/23/06.

"What lies behind you and what lies in front of you,

pales in comparison to what lies inside of you."

—Ralph Waldo Emerson

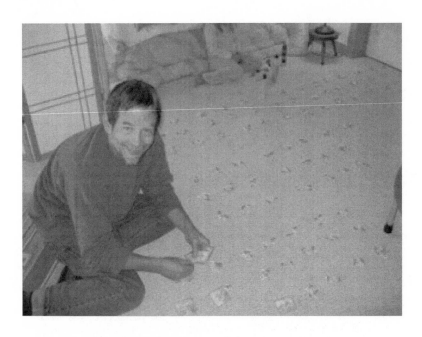

Laying out piles of daily supplements, 3/12/06.

ACKNOWLEDGEMENTS

Anne Stanton discovered our story while working as a reporter at the *Northern Express*. She implored us to write a book about our battle with cancer, and lovingly shepherded us though the first draft.

Anne Bardens-McClellan and Marcy Branski took their red pens to the manuscript and made invaluable suggestions.

Heather Shaw simply did the impossible. She made crucial editorial suggestions, created the book format and cover design, and helped us publish the book.

Last, but certainly not least, we would like to thank our family, friends, and patients for their love and support, both in our fight with cancer and in the writing of this book.

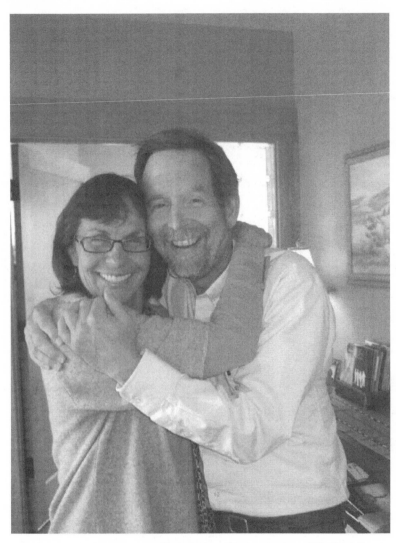

Photo by Anne Stanton courtesy of *Northern Express*

ABOUT THE AUTHORS

Greg Holmes, Ph.D. is a clinical psychologist in private practice in Traverse City . He has taught medical students and resident physicians in family medicine for over twenty years. His students have honored him with teaching awards for his contributions to their education. He is a popular speaker to the general public as well as the medical community.

Katherine Roth, M.D. is a board-certified family physician with thirty years of clinical experience. Prior to private practice, she worked as the associate director of the Family Medicine Residency Program at Sparrow Hospital in Lansing, Michigan. She currently works in private practice and is a much sought after expert in the field of integrative medicine.

Katherine and Greg have collaborated for over twenty years, educating physicians and caring for patients. During this time they have led support groups for patients with heart disease and cancer.

Made in the USA
Middletown, DE
28 July 2015